A-Z Herbal Remedies

Herbal remedies that have been used successfully for generations to treat numerous common ailments.

All rights reserved. No part of this book may be reproduced or utilized in any form or by any means, electronic or mechanical, including photocopying, recording or by any information storage and retrieval system, without permission in writing from the Publisher.

Table of Contents

Introduction 12
    Obtaining Herbs 16
    Preparation of Herbal Teas 19
1. Common Ailments and their Herbal Remedies 20
    Abscesses, Boils, Carbuncles 20
    Acidity 21
    Acne 22
    Adenoids 23
    Allergies 24
    Alopecia 24
    Anaemia 25
    Angina Pectoris 26
    Anorexia Nervosa 27
    Anxiety 28
    Appendicitis 29
    Appetite 29
    Arteriosclerosis 30
    Arthritis 31
    Asthma 34
    Athlete's Foot 35
    Backache 36

Bad Breath	36
Baldness	36
Bed-wetting	36
Biliousness	37
Bladder and Urinary Problems	38
Bleeding	38
Blood Disorders	38
Blood-Pressure	39
Boils and Carbuncles	40
Breast Feeding	41
Bronchitis	42
Bruises and Sprains	44
Burns and Scalds	44
Cancer	45
Carbuncles	46
Catarrh	46
Chilblains	48
Childrens' Ailments	48
Circulation	50
Coeliac Disease	50
Colic	51
Colitis	51
Common Colds and Chills	53
Conjunctivitis	54
Constipation	54

Convalescence 55

Corns 56

Coronary Thrombosis..56

Coughs 57

Cramp 58

Croup 59

Cystitis..59

Cysts 61

Dandruff..61

Deafness 61

Debility 62

Depression 63

Dermatitis 64

Diarrhoea 65

Digestive Disorders 65

Diverticulitis 67

Dizziness...68

Dropsy...68

Duodenal Ulcer 69

Dysentery 70

Dyspepsia 71

Ear Disorders..71

Eczema 72

Emphysema 73

Enteritis...73

Enuresis	74
Epilepsy	75
Erysipelas	75
Eye Problems	76
Fainting	77
Feet	78
Fevers	78
Fibrositis	79
Flatulence	79
Fractures	80
Freckles	81
Gallstones	81
Gastric Ulcer	82
Gastritis	83
Gastro-enteritis	84
Glandular Fever	85
Gout	86
Gravel	87
Gum and Mouth Problems	87
Haemorrhage	88
Haemorrhoids	89
Hair	90
Halitosis	90
Hay Fever	91
Heart Disorders	92

Heartburn	93
Hepatitis	93
Hernia	94
Hiccups	94
Hoarseness	95
Hyperactivity	95
Hypoglycaemia	95
Impetigo	97
Impotence	97
Incontinence	97
Infectious Disorders	98
Infertility	98
Inflammation	99
Influenza	100
Insect Bites and Stings	101
Insomnia	102
Irritable Bowel Syndrome	104
Jaundice	104
Kidney Disorders	105
Laryngitis	105
Lassitude	106
Lethargy	106
Liver	107
Lumbago	108
Lung Disorders	109

Lymphatic Glands 111

Malnutrition 111

Mastitis 112

Measles 112

Memory 113

Meniere's Disease 114

Menopause 115

Menstrual Disorders 117

Mental Fatigue 119

Migraine 119

Multiple Sclerosis 121

Nausea 121

Nervous Disorders 122

Nettle Rash 124

Neuritis and Neuralgia 125

Nightmares 126

Noises in the Ears 126

Nosebleed 126

Obesity 126

Osteomalacia 127

Osteoporosis 128

Pain 128

Palpitations 129

Pharyngitis 130

Phlebitis 130

Piles	131
Pleurisy	131
Polypus	132
Pregnancy and Childbirth	132
Prolapse	133
Prostate Gland	133
Pruritis	134
Psoriasis	135
Quinsy	136
Rheumatism	137
Rickets	139
Ringworm	139
Rupture	140
Sciatica	140
Sea-Sickness	141
Shingles	141
Shock	141
Sinusitis	142
Skin Problems	143
Sprains	145
Stomach Disorders	145
Stress	146
Strokes	147
Sunburn	147
Sunstroke	148

Swellings	148
Teething	149
Tension	149
Throat	150
Thrombosis	150
Tinnitus	151
Tonsillitis	152
Toothache	153
Travel Sickness	153
Tubercular Infection	154
Ulcers	155
Urinary Disorders	156
Uterine Disorders	157
Varicose Veins	158
Vertigo	159
Warts and Verrucas	160
Whitlow	160
Whooping Cough	160
Worms	161
Wounds	162
2. First Aid Box and Holiday First Aid	164
Holiday First Aid	165
3. Nutrition	167

Introduction

There is a rich age-old tradition of healing human ailments with wild plants, a tradition that has not died over thousands of years. The uses of healing plants have not varied, though today, with increasing knowledge of the origins of disease and of the pharmacology of plants, their uses have become better defined and understood. Herbs are a natural medicine, part of our inheritance.

An interest in plants may begin in childhood when we learn quickly to distinguish garden plants from weeds and may return from a walk in the country clutching a handful of wild flowers. Enlightened education may open our eyes to the profound wonder of plant life, and if we are more fortunate we may incorporate in this wonder an understanding of the medicinal uses of plants. We should make a study of plant remedies, although it must be said that the use of herbs is a skill and an art, and the most successful herbalist, in addition to studying intensively, must surely have some inherited gift of healing.

Plants draw sustenance from the soil and manufacture chlorophyll from sunlight. They contain many constituents: essential oils which give the plant its perfume and have medicinal properties (i.e., to aid digestion, to stimulate the nervous system, or if used as liniments, to increase the flow of blood to a given area); tannins, which have an astringent action on the mucosa; glycosides, some of which are anti-inflammatory, while some have -a regulating influence on heart action; mucilage's, which are used to soothe irritation and inflammation in the digestive tract; bitter principles which stimulate the secretion of digestive juices and improve the appetite. Numerous other constituents include resins, gums, minerals (notably sodium, potassium and silica), acids, vitamins and hormone precursors.

The herbal practitioner uses the total combination of these constituents, knowing that they will work in natural harmony together to have the desired influence on the body. The whole plant is used, or its roots, seeds or leaves, whichever part has the highest therapeutic value. The plant will be prepared in the form of tincture, liquid extract, syrup, tablet or external application, by methods which retain the optimum medicinal properties. Additionally, fresh or dried herbs are prescribed as tisanes or as fomentations.

Research in clinical laboratories and universities into the constituents of plants, seeking to isolate and then synthesize the most active substance has accelerated during the past decade or so. Isolation of the active principle has not always been so successful therapeutically as the researchers had hoped; it has been admitted that the single constituent has too harsh and powerful an action, whilst if administered in the complete plant form its action is controlled and assuaged. Warnings have been issued from time to time of the dangers of this or that plant. Investigation of the facts behind the warning reveal that massive doses of a single constituent have been administered to animals with unpleasant or fatal results, which should teach us that 'man can never excel nature in manufacturing medicines'.

Research by herbal practitioners and herbal manufacturers is not based on use of animals but on long-established usage, experience in practice hand-in-hand with modern pharmacological knowledge.

The increasing demand for herbal medicine continues unabated. What is its attraction? It is quite clear that more and more people are becoming disenchanted with modern drugs. Undoubtedly many of these can be life-savers, but they are often indiscriminately or carelessly used, and their side-effects can be numerous, often creating conditions that are as unpleasant and complex as the original disease they aim to treat. The side-effects of common drugs such as aspirin, which, if taken frequently can lead to peptic ulceration, or barbiturates which can deplete the nervous system, are giving rise to increasing concern. Hydrocortisone, so freely used to treat many inflammatory conditions from arthritis to skin disease, is destructive to the adrenal glands and can lead to the unpleasant disorder known as Cushing's syndrome, a disturbance which leads to weight increase and 'moonface' amongst other symptoms.

Anti-depressants and tranquillizers can initially give quick relief during illness, but often an increasing dose is required and attempts to discontinue the drugs after a while can give rise to a variety of symptoms more wretched than the original depression. The modern drugs relentlessly take their toll of our bodies, and taken alongside a diet of instant pre-packaged foods which are grown with artificial fertilizers and full of chemical additives, the natural vitality within us is sapped and drained.

In contrast to these potent and toxic drugs, a wealth of remedies that are effective and restorative is found in the healing plants, which exert a gentle action and bring about healing without suppressing symptoms. Used in the correct therapeutic dosages they are perfectly safe and without side-effects. Potentially toxic herbs are not used by the herbal practitioner, nor are they for sale. The isolates from plants that are used in orthodox medicine, such as digoxin from foxglove, are more dangerous than the whole plant remedy which contains other constituents to counteract and balance the action of the more potent ingredients. Two glycosides in *Convallaria majalis* (lily of the valley) have a stimulating and regulating effect on the heart muscle, very similar to the action of digoxin but without its cumulative properties. Other glycosides present in the plant have a diuretic effect and the total combination of constituents work in harmony. There has been no evidence, in hundreds of cases treated, that the action of *Convallaria* has caused over-stimulation or any abnormality of heart-rate, or had anything other than a beneficial effect on the heart.

It is used by the herbal practitioner for angina pectoris, to strengthen the ageing heart, and for conditions resulting from arteriosclerosis.

Regular use of herbs in salads and cooking can help to avoid many common ailments, and to build good health.

Familiar culinary herbs such as thyme, sage and rosemary, for example, are strongly antiseptic. Garlic is anticatarrhal, prevents worm-infestations, wards off colds and bronchitis and lowers blood cholesterol. In addition to the usual culinary herbs fresh plants such as dandelion leaves, chickweed, hawthorn leaves, fennel and lovage may be added to salads, enriching their nutritional and health giving properties. Infusions of herbs, taken regularly, will do much to improve and maintain health by their gentle action on different areas of the body. An infusion of chamomile or lemon balm taken after a meal for example, will enhance digestion, and calm and soothe the nervous system.

Dandelion root or leaf, taken as an infusion or decoction will improve liver function. A tea made of seeds such as fennel, caraway, anise and cardamom will help prevent flatulence after a heavy meal. Many herbal remedies with renowned medicinal properties owe much of their virtue to their rich content of minerals and vitamins. Nettles are a potent source of iron, silicon and potassium; dandelion root is rich in iron and potassium; rosehips are rich in vitamin C and bioflavonoids, coltsfoot contains zinc and horsetail silica.

Obtaining Herbs

Fresh herbs can be grown in your own garden, either from plants bought from a herb nursery or from wild-plant seeds from specialist suppliers. By growing the herbs one can be certain of having exactly the right plant. Small plants such as thyme and parsley can be grown in pots on a windowsill.

Some wild plants such as dandelion, nettles, plantain, coltsfoot, vervain, chamomile and agrimony could be allowed to grow in the garden if space allows.

Herbs may be gathered in the wild, but certain precautions must be taken. Make sure that they are free from insecticide sprays, traffic fumes and other chemicals, and that the plant is precisely the one that is wanted. Plants should be gathered only in wild, uncultivated places, away from roadsides and frequented canal or river banks. If there is any uncertainty about the plant a good botanical the plant should be dry (so do not gather in the early morning or late evening) and any withered leaves, damaged parts or insects should be discarded. Plants have periods in their life-cycle when their active constituents are at the optimum. This is normally when they are growing and reaching full growth, therefore plants should be collected just as they reach maturity. A patch of plants should be thinned, not cleared completely, so as to leave growth for subsequent years.

Rare or uncommon plants should never be gathered.

Flowers need to be gathered just as they have fully opened, and should be dried quickly away from sunlight.

Dry in the dark if the colour is to be preserved. Small flowers can be spread on paper, large ones hung in bunches in a dark, airy dry place.

Leaves are at their best when just at full maturity, a fresh, good green. The leaves, or the whole plant above ground if required, should be gathered just as the plant is on the point of flowering, and should be spread on clean paper, hessian or fine mesh trays, or hung in loose bunches away from sunlight and where the air can circulate, and should be turned or separated frequently.

Seeds should be gathered when ripe, spread out on clean paper and left for a few days.

Roots are at their best either in the spring or in the autumn. They should be cleaned of soil and chopped or sliced finely for drying either in sunlight or in the gentle heat in an oven. Large roots should be split lengthwise before chopping.

Plants which contain volatile oils should be gathered in the late afternoon of a sunny day, and should not be exposed to any heat whilst drying. They may be spread out and turned frequently or hung in small, loose bunches.

Herbs should be stored only in glass jars or in paper bags, not in plastic containers, and must be protected from light.

Aromatic plants especially should be stored carefully, as the volatile oils they contain are absorbed into plastic, rendering the plant much less useful. Dried herbs may be obtained from some health food stores and from a number of suppliers.

If something more sophisticated than herbal tea is desired, the many compounds and tablets available from health food stores and other suppliers will be found to be effective.

They are the result of practical experience with herbal medicine, and are produced in conformity with modern laboratory standards. The majority of the formulae have been prepared by practitioners for their patients during many successful years in practice.

This volume is not intended to replace professional attention, diagnosis and comprehensive treatment and is not a manual of totally independent self-treatment. If the condition to be dealt with is straightforward, then much can be done by using herbal remedies properly prepared in the form of infusions, decoctions or poultices. Herbal remedies used regularly at home may also be an adjunct in the case of more serious conditions, as they stimulate the body's defence mechanisms and accelerate the healing process. However, if there is any doubt about the condition, if it is serious or if there is no response to herbal tisanes, then help should be sought from a qualified practitioner.

Herbal practitioners

will be to seek and deal with the underlying cause of the problem, seeing the patient as a whole person and planning individual comprehensive treatment which will relieve the symptoms and leave the patient in much better general health.

Preparation of Herbal Teas

Unless stated otherwise in the text preparations and dosage of herbal teas are as follows:

Infusion: using leaves, flowers or whole herb apart from root or berries. Pour 1 pint (0.5 litres) of boiling water onto 1oz (25g) of finely chopped herb in a warmed vessel

Cover and leave to stand for fifteen minutes. Strain, keep in a covered vessel.

Decoction: using root, bark or berries. Add 1oz (25g) of the chopped or crushed remedy to 1 ½ pints (0.75 litres) of cold water, bring to the boil and simmer gently until reduced to 1pint (0.5 litre). Leave to cool, covered, then strain.

Dose: one wineglassful three times daily. A regular dose, approximately every eight hours, is the most effective.

It should be taken between meals unless advised differently in the text. A wineglassful is approximately three tablespoonfuls.

Herbal teas will keep for three to four days if kept, covered, in a refrigerator. If this is not possible a fresh supply should be made each day.

1. Common Ailments and their Herbal Remedies

Abscesses, Boils, Carbuncles

A sign of local infection, or a means of the body ridding itself of toxic wastes, an abscess must be encouraged to come to a head, to burst and to discharge its contents completely. This may be done by covering with a herbal poultice which will be changed at regular intervals, and by bathing with hot water when the poultice is changed.

Nettles boiled in just enough water to cover, applied hot and changed every eight hours, bathing with the hot liquid, are effective. Crushed or powdered fenugreek seeds mixed to a paste with hot milk, spread on cotton fabric and fixed firmly over the abscess will also draw it to a head, as will a poultice of castor oil. Powdered slippery elm, with a pinch of powdered capsicum added (a pinch to 1oz (25g») and mixed well, should be made into a paste with boiling water, quickly spread on the smooth side of lint and fastened firmly in place. This poultice should be changed every twentyfour hours. As a poultice, Abbott's No.1 paste can hardly be bettered. When the abscess is 'pointing' (coming to a head) bathe frequently with hot water and apply gentle pressure. Do not squeeze the abscess until it is ready to burst. Continue to apply slippery elm, as it will clear the abscess and also promote healing.

If abscesses or boils are recurrent, attention must be given to the general health by following a good diet rich in fresh raw salads, vegetables and fruits, poor in sugars, fats and starches. Herbal teas such as burdock root, fumitory, clivers and yellow dock root will be beneficial. An equal quantity of these, mixed well, is prepared by adding 1oz

(25g) to 1 1/2 pints (0.75 litre) of boiling water and simmering gently for fifteen minutes. Cool, strain and take a wineglassful three or four times daily. Echinacea herb is a good blood-purifier, and may be taken in wineglassful doses (the normal infusion), or is available in tablet form.

Acidity

Hyperacidity, an excessive production of the digestive acids in the stomach, is often associated with mental or emotional stress, and this aspect of health should be attended to (see Nervous Disorders, page 105). The finest herb for hyperacidity is meadowsweet, well named Queen of the Meadow. Infuse 1oz (25g) for twenty minutes in 1 pint (0.5 litre) of boiling water; a teacupful three times daily will help to correct acidity, and an extra dose may be taken at any time. Meadowsweet may be combined with an equal quantity of centaury herb and dandelion root, and 1oz (25g) of the mixed herbs to 1 pint (0.5 litre) prepared by simmering gently for fifteen minutes. A wineglassful should be taken after meals. Both peppermint tea and chamomile tea are useful. In addition papain tablets (made from the paw-paw fruit) help to neutralize stomach acid, and should be taken with meals. Gerard Papaya tablets include slippery elm and golden seal, both of which are soothing to the stomach and aid digestion.

The diet should be changed to include plenty of alkaline foods - salads, vegetable juices, green vegetables, carrots, and fruits such as sweet apples, grapes and pears. Pineapple contains enzymes which aid digestion, and the juice diluted with an equal quantity of warm water taken an hour after a meal will often give relief. Refined sugars and starches, sweets, jams, chocolate, alcohol, gooseberries, rhubarb, plums, tomatoes and spinach should all be excluded from the diet.

Acne

A skin problem in which the sebaceous glands of the skin become blocked and chronically inflamed, it is often due to the glandular changes which take place during adolescence, compounded by faulty diet. Nervous tension may be present and will aggravate the problem further. The herbal practitioner has a number of remedies which help the glandular disturbance, and will include echinacea, burdock root, dandelion root and red clover. These are mixed in equal quantities and 1oz (25g) of the mixture simmered gently for fifteen minutes in 1 1/2 pints (0.75 litre) of water; when cooled and strained a wineglassful should be taken three or four times daily. It may be advisable to add remedies for the liver and lymph glands. Blue flag root, poke root, barberry bark and chickweed are all valuable.

Attempts should be made to be more relaxed: tisanes of chamomile flowers or lime blossom will help, and an infusion of lavender (flowers, leaves and stalks) can be taken as a calming, soothing nerve remedy and also applied as lotion to oily skin. Add a handful of the fresh stalks or just under ½ oz (10g) of the flowers to 1 pint (0.5 litre) of boiling water, cover closely and leave to infuse for ten minutes. Strain, take a small teacupful morning and bedtime, and bathe the skin two or three times daily. Lotion or cream of marigold flowers is also good for oily skins, and infusion of elder flowers has been proved valuable as a skin tonic. Comfrey leaves infused for ten minutes, strained and cooled can be patted onto the skin for soothing and healing; an infusion of clivers herb used daily will cleanse the skin.

Do not squeeze the spots, maintain absolute cleanliness and avoid harsh perfumed soaps. Use very little make-up.

The diet should include plenty of fresh raw salads (especially watercress, parsley, young dandelion leaves and grated raw carrot every day), vegetables and fresh fruit; whole grains (whole-wheat, brown rice, etc.) and mixed proteins should replace sweets, chocolate, fried and fatty foods, white flour and white sugar products. Vitamin B complex, vitamin A and vitamin E are all necessary for a good healthy skin. Zinc tablets have been found to clear some cases of acne.

Wheat germ oil can be used to heal acne scars: snip a capsule and apply the oil. Used daily it will gradually promote healing.

Adenoids

The adenoids, like the tonsils, are part of the body's lymph gland defence system. They become enlarged and inflamed as a result of recurrent colds and catarrh. The herbal practitioner gives remedies which deal with the lymph glands and with catarrh, attending also to the general health. Provided a good diet is followed strictly, swollen adenoids can be reduced fairly quickly in most cases. Poke root and echinacea are especially useful (both are available' in tablet form) and reinforced by remedies for catarrh (see Catarrh, and Common Colds) should help to avoid the need for surgery. The child's general health must be considered; sweets, sugar, white flour products, refined breakfast cereals with added sugar, milk and milk products must all be avoided completely. Fresh fruit, unsweetened fruit juices, green vegetables and onions should be given in abundance. Plant milk or soya milk should replace cow's milk; dates and raisins may be eaten as sweets, and a little honey used for sweetening if necessary.

As a result of these changes catarrh normally clears up and the child's susceptibility to colds become much less.

Allergies

Hypersensitivity to a wide variety of substances. Dust, pollen, cat or dog hair, perfumes, wheat, milk and cheese are the most prominent of a long list. Allergic reactions include sudden recurrent 'colds', catarrh, watering eyes, skin rashes, diarrhoea, fatigue, poor sleep, irritability and, in children, restlessness, hyperactivity, mood swings, and sometimes learning difficulties. Avoiding the offending foods is only part of the answer, to overcome such hypersensitivity the herbal practitioner gives remedies to improve function of the liver, kidneys and digestion - dandelion root, centaury, vervain and fumitory for the liver, gentian root and calumba root to stimulate digestion.

A number of other remedies are used according to the individual patient's needs. Chamomile tea and peppermint tea can be of some assistance, but an allergic condition needs to be dealt with comprehensively. Persistence with herbal teas, coupled with a good diet, can overcome the allergic state. A raw-food diet is usually recommended. If this is not found possible the avoidance of processed foods which contain additives, and a high proportion of raw salads and vegetables could have a beneficial effect.

Alopecia

Loss of hair in patches on the scalp often indicates a reaction to stress or prolonged worry, and is reversible. General thinning of the hair can be due to hormonal changes, to drugs, or of course to advancing age. Herbal remedies, massage of the scalp, good nutrition and extra vitamins can lead to improvement. Clivers herb is rich in silica, a mineral the body needs for hair and nails; the normal infusion may be taken in wineglassful doses three times daily, and a little rubbed into the scalp daily. Nettles may be used in the same way, but a double-strength infusion should be prepared for external use. Rub it thoroughly into the scalp.

Nerve remedies can help, either herbal tisanes of lime blossom, skull cap or others, or herbal nerve tablets (Heath & Heather, or Roberts, for example).

General health should be considered, a good diet supplemented by vitamin B complex, vitamin A, vitamin C (at least 500mg daily), one kelp tablet daily, and at least two teaspoonfuls of molasses each day.

Advice should be sought for this problem if the above measures have no effect.

Anaemia

Anaemia may be either a reduction in the number of red blood cells in the bloodstream, or a lack of haemoglobin (the red pigment in blood which carries iron). The red blood cells carry oxygen from the lungs to all parts of the body, the oxygen combining with iron to form haemoglobin; a lack of either oxygen or iron leads to debility, headaches, faster heartbeat and a general feeling of malaise. Anaemia may be due to obvious blood loss such as haemorrhage or heavy menstruation, it may be secondary to some other illness, be due to a failure of bone marrow to produce new cells, or to the body's inability to assimilate sufficient iron from food. A cause which must not be overlooked is drug treatment for some other condition. The herbal practitioner deals with the problem by giving remedies to improve digestion and assimilation, supplemented by herbal alternatives which improve the quality of blood, by attending to any other health problems and by ensuring a good diet is followed. A valuable herbal drink is prepared from equal quantities of dandelion root, nettles, vervain, marigold flowers and comfrey leaves. Allow *1oz* (12.5g) of each to stand in 3 pints (1.5 litres) of cold water for one hour, then bring to the boil, keep at boiling point for five minutes then simmer down to 2 pints (1 litre). Strain when cool, and take a wineglassful half an hour before each meal. A tea of either hops or bog bean taken in wineglassful doses after meals will help the body assimilate iron. If tablets are preferred, Roberts' *An-em* tablets will be found helpful.

Certain herbs contain iron and should be included in the diet: parsley, nettles, alfalfa, elderberries, also blackberries, blackcurrants, chickweed and watercress. Elderberries are laxative if taken in large quantities. Nettles can be cooked as spinach, and be taken as an extra iron-rich vegetable.

Whole grains, oats, millet, brown rice, molasses, black treacle, raisins, figs, prunes and apricots stewed together, dates, black grapes, onions and green leafy vegetables should be taken in abundance. Almonds, Brazil nuts, sunflower seeds, lentils and above all soya beans will provide iron, calcium and other necessary minerals.

Needless to say, professional advice must be sought if no improvement takes place.

Angina Pectoris

An intense pain in the chest together with a feeling of pressure or suffocation, always occurring on exertion, is usually caused by spasmodic contraction of blood vessels inhibiting oxygen supply to the heart. The pain quickly eases on rest. It may also be the result of spinal vertebrae being slightly out of alignment. It is commonly associated with tension and anxiety, and is not entirely a disease of the heart and circulation.

One of the remedies for angina is the familiar hedgerow tree, hawthorn. An infusion of the flowers (one teaspoonful to a teacupful of boiling water) will beneficially influence blood vessels, gradually strengthen and correct the heart action, and will slowly lower high blood-pressure to the individual's normal level. A teacupful of either the flower infusion or a decoction of the berries may be taken two or three times daily for long periods without any hazard. The decoction is made by simmering *1 oz* (12.5g) of the berries in 2 pints (1 litre) of water for five minutes. Hawthorn is also available in tablet form.

A diet which is almost completely vegetarian and free from animal fats and salt helps greatly. Reduction of weight if necessary, avoidance of worry and adequate relaxation will contribute to overcoming this disorder.

Garlic lowers blood-pressure and reduces blood cholesterol, so could be a good adjunct to the measures recommended above. Two garlic oil capsules or garlic and parsley tablets taken regularly at bedtime will suffice.

Anorexia Nervosa

A problem in which the majority of sufferers are young Women between the ages of fifteen and twenty-three.

There may be organic disease present, but the main cause of the disorder appears to be psychological. A wide range of theories, from subconscious rejection of sexual maturity to family and emotional pressures, have been put forward but no single theory is totally convincing.

Anorexics need expert help and so a practitioner with some ability in positive Natural Psychotherapy should be sought. A number of remedies are prescribed by the herbal practitioner, including centaury and agrimony for the liver and appetite, with nervines such as skull cap, passion flower and chamomile flowers. The combination of centaury, gentian root, agrimony and skull cap herb, 102 (25g) of the mixture simmered gently for ten minutes in 1pint (0.5 litre) of water, taken in wineglassful doses three or four times daily, will promote appetite. A pinch of powdered cinnamon added to the herbal teas will reinforce their action, but much more than simple herbal teas is usually needed in the treatment of this condition.

Anxiety

A state of worrying about anything and everything, associated with tight breathing, palpitations, perspiration and a variety of other symptoms. Herbal medicine can be very helpful in this condition, combined with good nutrition

(especially supplements of vitamin B complex and calcium) and some exploration of background causes of the anxiety state. Relaxation exercises plus plenty of yawning and stretching will help to break the pattern of muscular tension.

Herbal teas taken regularly, three times daily with an occasional extra wineglassful when required, will gradually bring about improvement.

Wood betony alone or combined with equal quantities of hyssop, skull cap and lime flowers will make a good start.

Take 1oz (25g) of the mixture, add to 1 pint (0.5 litre) of boiling water with a little honey or liquorice to sweeten if desired. This combination will promote some relaxation, thus relieving some of the tension. The wood betony and lime blossom will help to calm the mind at bedtime, leading to a better night's sleep (see also Insomnia).

There are many herbal mixtures and tablets which will be found helpful, Roberts' Nerfood tablets, Heath &Heather's nerve tablets and Napier's nerve tablets.

Anxiety may be a life-long problem, the tendency being acquired during childhood from anxious parents, and it will be necessary to persist with the treatment for some months.

Appendicitis

Acute appendicitis must be treated promptly and correctly to avoid the danger of a burst appendix and peritonitis. It should not be treated by the inexperienced.

Prevention is the criterion, by having a high-fibre diet thus keeping the bowels functioning regularly with a bulky stool. If warning symptoms of acute appendicitis develop, the sufferer should fast on water only until the temperature has returned to normal, and hot fomentations should be applied over the painful area - either plain hot water or an infusion of elderflowers. Occasionally niggling pains in the right side of the abdomen are described as a grumbling appendix. Garlic capsules should be taken regularly to deal with this, and the diet should consist of fresh raw fruits, home-made vegetable soups and natural yogurt. The bowels must be encouraged to open freely. If the diet is insufficient for this, ten to twenty drops of extract of cascara in warm water with a tiny pinch of powdered ginger should be taken each night, or an enema of one to two pints taken daily. Extract of cascara should be obtainable from a good chemist, or from a herbal supplier.

Appetite

It is natural to lose appetite during acute illness. Fasting on fruit juices or pure water is the right way to help the body to rid itself as quickly as possible of the infection. Appetite returns naturally when the body is ready to cope with food, and is one of the good signs during convalescence.

A number of herbs used as tonics will stimulate the appetite at such a time, but should not be given during the acute stage. An infusion of agrimony herb is a good tonic and stimulant, but as it is astringent should not be given when constipation is present. A decoction of gentian root will influence the liver and digestion, will promote appetite and aid the assimilation of food. Take two teaspoonfuls before meals. It is very bitter, even when diluted. Poplar bark is also an excellent tonic, useful during convalescence and debility, aiding appetite and digestion. The following recipe will help: take 1oz (25g) each of gentian root, agrimony herb, centaury and calumba root, allow to stand for half an hour in 2 pints (1 litre) of cold water, then bring to the boil and simmer gently for five minutes. Take a wineglassful, slightly warm, one hour before each meal.

Peppermint tea taken two or three times daily will improve the appetite.

Arteriosclerosis

Hardening and thickening of the walls of arteries, associated with deposits of cholesterol on the inner surfaces, often precedes coronary thrombosis, and is therefore a condition to be prevented as far as possible and dealt with promptly when discovered. Hardened arteries, when not an inherited condition, are the result of many years of wrong diet - refined carbohydrates, animal fats and convenience foods in abundance, a deprivation of vitamins B, C and E, lecithin, whole grains, fresh fruit, salad and vegetables.

Research into the action of garlic has shown that it helps control the cholesterol content of the blood and plays a part in reducing, to some extent, the fatty deposits inside blood vessels. Use garlic in cooking and take three garlic oil capsules at bedtime every night.

Lime blossom, hawthorn and nettles are all excellent remedies for arteriosclerosis, and may be taken alone or in combination. Lime blossom tea is sedative and antispasmodic, tending to 'thin' the blood, thus reducing blood-pressure in the hardened arteries. Prepare it by adding half a teaspoonful of dried flowers, chopped finely, to a teacupful of boiling water, covering closely and leaving to cool. Drink this between meals twice daily. Hawthorn contributes to dissolving the deposits on the inner surface of blood vessels, strengthening and regulating the heart's action, reducing blood-pressure by dilating blood vessels and by its sedative action on the nervous system (see Angina) for directions on its preparation). Nettles will also, gradually, reduce the cholesterol deposits and will strengthen the arteries. Add 1oz (25g) of chopped leaves and stalks to 2 pints (1 litre) of boiling water. Simmer gently for five minutes. Allow to cool for ten minutes, strain and take a wineglassful three times daily.

Combine regular herbal teas with a good diet, as indicated above.

Arthritis

A form of rheumatism in which the inflammation is limited to joints, affecting the cartilages, ligaments and other tissues controlling joint movement, and the bones themselves.

It can be divided clinically into two main types: rheumatoid arthritis, a systemic disease affecting many joints throughout the body, and osteo-arthritis which occurs only in weight-bearing joints. The condition can be less clear-cut, in that both types may be present at the same time, or some other disease may be running concurrently and altering the development of the arthritis. It also occurs in other forms: Still's disease, arthritis of childhood; ankylosing spondylitis in which the spine becomes rigid; Reiter's disease, and various types of arthritis which are the result of some infection, trauma or from menopausal hormone changes. There is, in many cases, a background of long-standing emotional tensions, which alone can alter hormone production and subsequently affect assimilation of food. Faulty nutrition contributes much to the cause.

Correct diagnosis is essential; self-treatment can be inadequate unless it is allied with practitioner care.

The herbal practitioner uses a number of herbs in treating arthritis, including in his formula whichever ones are specifically indicated for the individual case. One of the most useful herbs is meadowsweet, used for its antacid and sedative properties. Corn silk is used particularly to reduce the uric acid level, as is gravel root, prickly ash often added to the formula to improve the circulation. Sarsaparilla, burdock root, bogbean, black cohosh, and above all celery seed are combined in differing quantities. A number of excellent herbal mixtures or tablets are available, and can be taken with safety. Celery seed tablets are a first necessity, and could be reinforced in their action by

Robert's Prickly Ash Compound, one of Heath & Heather's mixtures or by Devil's Claw tablets.

Self-help can take several forms: good nutrition; vitamin therapy; exercise; good posture, and a positive mental approach. Arthritis sufferers have been found to have a low level of vitamins C, B complex and E. Drugs given in the treatment of arthritis deplete the body of its vitamins, especially C and B. Long-sustained stress causes over activity of the adrenal glands, which require vitamin C for healthy functioning. Vitamin C is also needed to build strong collagen tissue around the joints and to help the body assimilate calcium. At least two grams of vitamin C (from rose-hip or acerola cherry), 200IU vitamin E, four B complex and one vitamin A capsule should be taken daily.

A lacto-vegetarian diet is advisable, and should include lots of celery and parsley, fresh green vegetables, whole grains, sunflower and sesame seeds and home-made vegetable soups. Sugars and starches, animal fats, red meat and alcohol should be kept to the minimum. Citrus fruits, gooseberries, rhubarb and plums are best avoided as the majority of arthritics experience aggravation of the pain after eating them. Conversely, relief has been found when taking a teaspoonful of cider vinegar in warm water, with a little honey to taste. It may be taken first thing in the morning or just before meals to correct deficient production of digestive acids. Exercise should be sufficient to keep the joints mobile, but not so much as to cause fatigue. Walking, swimming and yoga are the most suitable.

Daily relaxation can help, especially in rheumatoid arthritis which is often associated with emotional trauma, unresolved conflicts and chronic resentment.

Tea and coffee are best avoided, and can be replaced by parsley or celery seed tea (a teaspoonful of either in a teacupful of boiling water, covered, cooled and strained), vegetable juices and Vecon. Vichy water will reduce acidity and aid digestion by increasing enzyme production, and if taken hot it will assist bowel action.

Asthma

There will be no success in the treatment of asthma by only paying attention to relieving symptoms. It is essential that the causes are dealt with adequately and the general health is improved. The asthmatic child is often a highly-strung, nervous and sensitive individual, with perhaps an hereditary predisposition to asthma. There may be an early history of recurrent colds and catarrh and possibly some eczema.

Asthma is associated with under-activity of the adrenal glands, sluggish function of the kidneys and some irritability of the nervous system. Faulty diet, such as one which allows high intake of milk and sugary foods, also contributes to the problem.

The herbal practitioner will give a combination of expectorants to aid in clearing the lungs - these would include hyssop, coltsfoot, mullein, comfrey, grindelia and mallow, and he would also recommend garlic. Remedies will be given to soothe nervous irritability and sensitivity. Hops, skull cap, chamomile flowers and lime blossom are useful.

A helpful regime (although asthma needs the help of a herbal practitioner and perhaps osteopathic manipulation to relieve upper thoracic tension) would be to take garlic capsules at bedtime and a herbal tea during the day. This could comprise equal quantities of comfrey leaves, hyssop, coltsfoot, chamomile and skull cap. Mixed well, 1 oz (25g) should be simmered gently for five minutes in 1 pint (0.5 litre) of water, then strained through a fine cloth or paper coffee filter. The dose would be a wineglassful three times daily for an adult, and half the dose for a child. (The age definition should be about fifteen years, depending on the child's weight.) A daily hot bath which contains catmint or pine would help, taken at bedtime.

Deep slow breathing must be practised daily. Learn abdominal breathing and breathe *out* as long and as slowly. as possible. This breathing can then be attempted to ease an asthma attack. Place the hands across the abdomen below the ribs and breathe in, feeling the abdomen being pushed out. Hold for a moment then breathe out slowly. Do not force the lungs too full, the accent is on breathing out. An attack may also be alleviated by hot and cold compresses over the upper chest, or by a hot foot bath. A teaspoonful of honey, in which finely sliced garlic has been steeped, taken in a cup of hot water and sipped slowly may also relieve an attack.

Diet should include plenty of raw salads, onions, green vegetables, and should exclude refined sugar and flour, milk (even skimmed or powdered milk) and fatty, fried foods.

Athlete's Foot
Strict hygiene is necessary to get rid of this fungal infection which settles between the toes. The infection is often picked up at swimming baths and gymnasiums.

Take care to wash and dry the feet thoroughly, especially between the toes. Apply tincture of myrrh or cider vinegar, diluting it a little if the skin is broken. Apply at least twice daily. Footbaths can help; one recommended by Kitty

Little consists of1oz (25g) each of red clover, sage, marigold flowers and agrimony herb simmered gently for twenty minutes in 5/4 pints (3 litres) of water. Strain, using the herbs as poultices between the toes. Add two teaspoonfuls of cider vinegar to the liquid when it has cooled to a comfortable temperature. Bathe the feet in this liquid for half an hour, and then dry thoroughly. Powder between the toes with arrowroot. Regular use of both footbath and lotion will eventually overcome the infection.

Backache

The cause must be diagnosed; it may be simple back strain, bad posture, kidney infection or disease, or uterine problems, to mention but a few. Bad posture can be corrected by a practitioner who teaches the Alexander technique, an osteopath will correct a misaligned spinal column, and strained back muscles will respond to rest, warmth and massage. Rub two or three times daily with a good herbal oil or liniment. A simple oil may be prepared by covering fresh, clean, dry St John's Wort herb with olive oil and heating it very gently (in a stainless steel pan) until the plant has lost its fresh green colour and is beginning to feel very slightly crisp. Filter the oil when cool. Oil which contains wintergreen will also be useful. Many herbal practitioners have their own formulated rubbing oils; others are available from health food stores.

Taking Roberts' Buchu Backache Compound, Heath &

Heather's backache tablets or similar remedies will speed up relief.

Bad Breath (see Halitosis)

Baldness (see Alopecia)

Bed-wetting (see Enuresis)

Biliousness

The simple bilious disorder which results from over-eating rich foods is easily overcome by fasting for twenty-four hours, or until the symptoms have subsided completely, and by drinking infusions of peppermint or chamomile tea every two hours. Both of these herbs help to relieve nausea and headaches and are relaxing to the nervous system.

Mint tea, made from the common garden mint *(Mentha spicata and M. rotundifolia),* affords the same benefits, but should not be taken by nursing mothers as breast milk will be diminished.

Recurrent biliousness must be dealt with more thoroughly, by taking herbal teas three times daily for some months and by amending the diet. Gentian root taken in tablespoonful doses three times daily before meals will help improve the digestion and will influence liver function. It is rather bitter, so a small quantity of mint or lime blossom could be added to the preparation to alter the flavour a little. Steep ½ oz (12.5g) of finely chopped gentian root in 1 pint (0.5 litre) of cold water for fifteen minutes.

Bring to the boil and simmer very gently for ten minutes, adding the mint or lime blossom at the end of the time.

Cool, then strain. Alternatively, one of the prepared mixtures for the liver and digestion could be very helpful, for example Roberts' Nervous Dyspepsia tablets.

Avoid fried foods, reduce fats, dairy produce, chocolate and all sweet foods to the minimum.

Bladder and Urinary Problems

A large number of herbs can be used to relieve the simple problems which arise from time to time. Both divers and gravel root are relaxing and soothing to the kidneys, helping to promote the flow of urine, may be used together or alone. Gravel root, as its name implies, issued by the herbal practitioner to eliminate urinary deposits from the kidneys.

Marshmallow root contains mucilage which is very soothing to the mucous membrane lining of bladder and urinary system. A decoction is valuable in any inflammatory or irritated state, such as cystitis or urethritis. Buchu leaves are wonderfully beneficial to the urinary system, stimulating but not irritating, increasing the quantity of urine secreted, relieving an aching back. In hot infusion it soothes the pelvic nerves and mucous membranes of the urinary system. Two tablespoonfuls of the normal infusion should be taken three times daily. Buchu is included in Potter's

Antitis tablets, and is available also in tablet form from other suppliers. Uva ursi herb is helpful to most bladder and urinary problems; a wineglassful of the normal infusion should be taken three times daily.

Follow a sensible diet, avoiding coffee, tomatoes and spinach and eating plenty of carrots. An infusion of fresh carrot tops will be found to be very helpful.

See also Urinary Disorders.

Bleeding (see Haemorrhage)

Blood Disorders

The traditional herbalist's remedies of a 'spring tonic' were badly needed after a winter's diet of stodgy foods and lack of fresh raw foods; a crop of boils, skin eruptions, a coated tongue, bad breath and constipation signalled the need for good herbal 'blood purifiers'. An excellent combination is equal quantities of burdock root, red dover flowers, divers, fumitory, bog bean and dandelion root. Make sure that the roots are chopped finely so as to yield their properties. Mix well, and add 2 oz (50g) to 2 pints (1 litre) of cold water bring to the boil and simmer gently for fifteen minutes. Cover and leave to cool, strain and take a wineglassful three times daily. These herbs will influence the liver and kidneys, aiding natural removal of impurities. Echinacea tablets may also be taken, more particularly for skin eruptions. Young dandelion leaves, parsley, watercress and celery added to the daily salad will accelerate the action of the herbal remedies.

Blood poisoning, from a bite or injury, needs urgent and professional attention. If not available, fasting on pure water and fruit juices, with doses every two or three hours of the above herbal tea, alternating with echinacea tablets, should be effective. Poultices applied to the original bite could be helpful (see Abscesses).

Blood-Pressure

High

Causes of high blood-pressure must be sought. There may be kidney or heart disease, hardened arteries, 'nerves', dietary faults, or there may be no obvious cause.

Garlic has been proved to lower blood-pressure and to reduce the cholesterol content of the blood, and it is therefore one of the most useful remedies to use. A clove of garlic daily, chopped finely and mixed with food will work wonders (although not for your social life!).

Alternatively, two or three garlic oil capsules taken at bedtime will be almost as effective. Herbal teas such as lime blossom, hawthorn, nettle or yarrow will lower blood pressure caused by nervous tension; a wineglassful of the normal infusion should be taken three times daily. Gerard

Hawthorn tablets, Roberts' BP tablets, Weleda Avena sativa compound, or other prepared remedies which may be obtained from the health food store will, if taken regularly and combined with good nutrition, lower high blood-pressure which is the result of normal causes. Diet should be amended to include lots of green leafy vegetables, raw salads, onions (raw or cooked) and fresh fruits, and should exclude animal fats, fried foods, alcohol, coffee and strong tea. Dandelion coffee, Mate, Luaka or Rooibosch tea, apple and grape juices may all be taken as beverages which are both pleasant and therapeutic.

Low
Lower than average blood-pressure can be normal to an individual for most of his life without there being anything wrong, but a change in a person's normal blood-pressure which occurs other than after an illness should be investigated.

Ginseng, acting as a tonic to all systems of the body, will in most cases gradually raise blood-pressure to its normal level. It is a remedy which is slow in action, and needs to be taken for some months to gain full benefit, then stopped for a couple of months. The herbal practitioner has a number of remedies which are pr

Boils and Carbuncles (see Abscesses)

Breast Feeding

An infant who has been breast-fed for the first six months of life will have greater resistance to infection than one who has not, and the longer the breast-feeding continues the stronger the child will be. Herbs have been used throughout the ages, both to help promote the supply of milk and to dry it up when weaning has been completed.

The herbs which help promote milk supply (and obviously will not harm the baby) are milkwort, fenugreek seeds, borage, holy thistle and dill. Normal infusion of the milkwort should be taken in wineglassful doses two or three times daily. An ounce (25g) of the crushed fenugreek seeds should be simmered gently for two minutes in 1pint (0.5 litres) of water, and a small cupful of both liquid and seeds taken at least twice daily. The same preparation can be taken during the pregnancy as general strengtheners' and tonic. The normal infusion of borage should be taken in wineglassful doses night and morning. Holy thistle has a bitter taste and honey should be added to the normal infusion. Take a small teacupful night and morning. Both borage and holy thistle will be useful against postnatal depression.

If it is necessary to dry up the milk supply an infusion of periwinkle herb, or of mint, taken in wineglassful doses three times daily will have the desired effect. Distilled witch-hazel applied to the nipples will clear up seepage of milk. Weleda calendula ointment is soothing for sore or cracked nipples. Do not take garlic when breast-feeding, as it will cause the baby to have digestive upsets.

Bronchitis

A cold which settles on the chest or an attack of acute bronchitis with its sudden feeling of rawness and oppression in the chest, raised temperature and aching limbs, should both be treated promptly and thoroughly and the body's natural resistance be built up so as to prevent the onset of chronic bronchitis.

In the early stages perspiration should be encouraged with hot drinks of yarrow tea, elderflower and peppermint (with composition essence added if there is a feeling of chilliness), or hyssop and horehound together. Any of them should be taken in wineglassful doses every hour and should prevent the condition from worsening. No food should be taken, only drinks of lemon juice in hot water sweetened with honey. If a cough develops add marshmallow root and liquorice root to the hyssop and horehound. Use equal quantities of each, 1 oz (25g) of the mixture added to 2 pints (1 litre) of cold water, brought to the boil and simmered gently for five minutes. This can be taken in wineglassful doses several times daily. Garlic is a fine antiseptic, useful for both acute and chronic bronchitis. Two large cloves of garlic should be sliced finely, added to 4oz (100g) of liquid honey and left, covered, to stand overnight. A teaspoonful of this honey in a half-teacupful of hot water will soothe a troublesome cough. Onion can be used in the same way.

Garlic should not be taken by nursing mothers.

Chronic bronchitis may need the attention of a practitioner to give massage or manipulation, advice on diet and on breathing exercises and to provide specific medicine. The chronic condition usually occurs in middle life, often after many years of chesty colds, damp climate or work in a dusty atmosphere.

Comfrey will be found to be a useful remedy in chronic bronchitis, its demulcent properties soothing irritated bronchial passages. Use the root, allowing 4oz (100g) of finely sliced root to stand for four hours in 2 pints (1 litre) of tepid water. Strain the liquid and take a wineglassful three times daily.

Another remedy for long-term use is grindelia, valuable for both chronic bronchitis and bronchial asthma. Prepare by adding one teaspoonful of the leaves and flowers, a small stick of liquorice (chopped) and a pinch of anise seeds to a teacupful of boiling water. Cover, leave to infuse for fifteen minutes, strain and drink in dessertspoonful doses during the day. Many other herbs can be used, and are included in the various preparations available from the health food stores or from individual herbal suppliers. The practitioner will dispense an individual formula for each patient, according to that patient's specific condition.

The long-term treatment of chronic bronchitis requires good nutrition to support herbal remedies. Milk in all forms should be avoided, with the exception of plant milk or soya milk. The diet should consist mostly of fresh raw fruits, salads and vegetables, mixed proteins with a low percentage of animal protein, whole-wheat bread and crisp bread in small quantities and plenty of fruit juices to drink. Strong tea, coffee and alcohol should be avoided.

Fasting on fruit juices and appropriate herbal teas is the most effective way of dealing with an attack of bronchitis.

The chest should be rubbed each night with Olbas oil or similar, so that the valuable fumes are inhaled during sleep.

Bruises and Sprains

Several herbs are excellent: apply a pad of lint, cotton wool or cotton fabric soaked in any of the following: distilled witch hazel, diluted tincture of arnica (two teaspoonfuls to a teacupful of cold water), an infusion of comfrey leaves, marigold flowers or hyssop herb, or comfrey oil. Bind the compress firmly in place, but not so tightly as to impede circulation. Keep the pad moist with the selected remedy, and continue until after all the swelling or tenderness has cleared. The herbal infusions for this purpose are made by barely covering the herb with boiling water and leaving to cool. If comfrey oil is available apply it immediately, keeping a bandage moistened with the oil fastened around the injury.

Burns and Scalds

Whatever is available of the following remedies will soothe and heal normal burns and scalds. Apply with clean fingertips or soak clean cotton fabric and cover gently. Do not apply cotton wool or the fluffy side of lint, as these will dry and stick to the injured skin.

Comfrey oil, elder leaves oil, crushed elderberries; elderflower infusion, distilled witch hazel, an infusion of blackberry leaves, marshmallow leaves or St John's Wort, honey or even cabbage leaves. The cabbage should be fresh, the leaf washed then pounded to make it soft and soaked for half an hour in just enough olive oil to cover it. The soft leaf and oil are then applied to the burn. Elder or comfrey leaves can be prepared in the same way for emergency use.

Honey can be spread thinly on cotton fabric and changed every twelve hours.

Major Burns and scalds, covering large areas of the body, must have professional medical attention, but until that help arrives cover the area with clean cotton cloths soaked in tepid water and keep the cloths cool. Give treatment for shock.

Cancer

No recommendation is given here for herbal treatment of cancer; the disease needs comprehensive professional treatment. Old herbals refer to remedies for tumours and swellings, and current research is finding anti-tumour properties in many plants, but self-treatment must not be undertaken.

Concern should lie with preventive measures, avoiding the known carcinogens, the substances in everyday life which are experimentally and statistically associated with cancer: tobacco, nitrates and other preservatives in tinned meats, sausages, etc., sweeteners, mineral oil and coal tar products, food dyes, many of the food additives used so freely to flavour, preserve and emulsify modern foods, and many, many other substances used in industry, medicine and cosmetics. Each carcinogen taken alone in minute quantities can be tolerated by the body without hazard, but if the body's vitality is lowered by stress, virus infection or other illness, its ability to cope will be so much reduced that the cumulative effect of numerous carcinogens even in the tiniest amounts over a period of time could lead to the occurrence of random cellular abnormalities of the type which develop into tumours.

Herbal remedies taken regularly to maintain good health, vitality and efficient functioning of the liver and kidneys, coupled with a wholesome diet of fresh foods free from artificial fertilizers and toxic sprays should do much to ward off the disease. There should be adequate protein but not too much, and avoidance of refined, denatured and processed foods which give little to the body but calories and artificial flavours. At least half the foods should be raw: fresh sun-ripened fruits, fresh salads with a simple dressing of lemon juice, oil and herbs, fresh organically-grown vegetables. Dr Bircher-Benner, the renowned doctor and nutritionist claimed that in order to maintain good health fifty per cent of the food eaten should be raw; if ill the raw food should be increased to seventy-five per cent, and if seriously ill all foods should be raw and a vegetarian diet followed.

The patient should be encouraged to take an active role in endeavouring to restore health, using strict dieting, relaxation, visual imagery and other methods of alternative treatment which could be used in conjunction with whatever treatment the patient was undertaking. Within a short time demand for help increased tremendously, and aroused wide interest in the medical profession. This approach accords with the herbal practitioner's principles of treating the patient as a whole being and supporting the body's own healing forces.

Carbuncles (see Abscesses)

Catarrh

Inflammation of the sensitive mucous membrane lining of nasal passages, throat and sinuses leads to an increased production of mucus, which in the healthy state is secreted to protect and moisten the area. In colds and other infections it is the body's way of ridding itself of toxins, as is the case in chronic catarrh.

Many herbs can be used to overcome catarrh in combination with strict dieting. Garlic should be eaten whenever possible, sliced and steeped in honey (see Bronchitis, for details) and two garlic oil capsules taken at bedtime. Herbal teas of equal quantities of yarrow, boneset, eyebright, white horehound and sage, 1oz (25g) of the mixture infused for twenty minutes in 1 pint (0.5 litre) of boiling water, strained and taken in half-teacupful doses four or five times daily will gradually clear catarrh. If the catarrh is affecting the chest, 1oz (25g) of a mixture comprising marshmallow leaves, white horehound and centaury added to 1 1/2 pints (0.75 litre) of cold water, brought to the boil and simmered gently for fifteen minutes, strained and taken three times daily in wineglassful doses, will soothe and help clear the catarrh. Hyssop tea, normal preparation and dose, will help clear the mucus and will soothe the irritated passages. Agrimony herb is a good astringent, influencing mucous membrane tissues. Taken in wineglassful doses three times daily it is valuable for chronic catarrh or catarrh following influenza, when it will help stimulate the appetite. Because of its astringency it has a good effect on loose bowel action, but is not advised in constipation. There are a number of proprietary remedies for catarrh: Potter's Antifect; Roberts' Catarrh tablets;

Heath & Heather's nasal catarrh mixture and others. Oil of Eucalyptus, Abbott's nasal oil, Olbas oil or similar herbal preparation should be used daily as an inhalant, and a little sprinkled on the pillow at bedtime to be inhaled whilst sleeping.

Milk and its products should be eliminated from the diet, plenty of onions, raw salads, vegetables and fresh fruits should be included. Lemon and grapefruit juices in hot water on rising and at bedtime will help clear the catarrh, and one day each week on these alone, no food at all, will be beneficial in chronic catarrh. Vitamin C is a good supplement; take at least 500mg daily.

Chilblains

Due to poor circulation, chilblains should be treated by a combination of applications to ease the itching and soreness, herbal teas to improve the circulation and to strengthen blood vessels, by exercise and by improved diet.

For unbroken chilblains, tincture of myrrh, lemon juice or distilled witch-hazel applied several times daily will reduce the inflammation. If the skin is broken apply honey, marshmallow ointment or calendula cream. Bathe the feet or hand for ten minutes twice daily in a warm infusion of marigold flowers (the normal infusion), alternating with plain cold water, three minutes in the warm infusion, half a minute in the cold, repeating six times.

Take buckwheat tea, rutin tablets, or a tea prepared by adding one teaspoonful each of crushed hawthorn berries, chopped angelica root and yarrow to 1/2 pint (0.25 litres) of boiling water, covering and allowing to cool. Strain, and take a wineglassful three times daily. This should not be taken by diabetics unless the angelica is omitted. Roberts' 'Drops of Life' mixture is useful. Take a brisk walk each day, swim, cycle, do energetic arm and leg exercises several times daily.

See also Circulation.

Childrens' Ailments

Children can be treated with perfect safety, the doses of herbal infusions being given as follows:

age 10 to 14 years - half adult dose (one tablespoonful)

age 6 to 10 years - one dessertspoonful

age 2 to 6 years - two to three teaspoonfuls

an infant up to 2 years - one teaspoonful

Raspberry leaves are excellent for soothing and toning small children and infants, and can be used for diarrhoea, stomach upsets and for sore mouths; give warm for a chill or cold. Add the teaspoonful dose to the bottle feed if this is the most convenient method.

For infants' digestive upsets dill water or aniseed will help. Add one teaspoonful of anise seeds (crushed) to a teacupful of boiling water, cover and leave to cool- strain.

Give a teaspoonful before each feed.

For childrens' diarrhoea, a normal infusion of agrimony herb, or blackberry leaves, will soon control the condition.

Give the dose according to age, three or four times daily.

Colds and fevers respond quickly to warm drinks of catmint herb, lemon balm or chamomile flowers. Add a little lemon juice and honey.

Vague aches and pains will be relieved by a warm infusion of catmint. If stomach pains do not respond to this, antispasmodic tincture, peppermint tea or chamomile tea should be tried. If the pains still do not ease seek the help of a practitioner.

Nappy rash can be soothed by elderflower ointment, and infantile eczema is often cleared by We1eda Sambucus comp.

Antispas is a fine remedy for all ages; a few drops in the feed of an infant will resolve many digestive problems, and a half-teaspoonful in warm water or milk and water will benefit an older child.

The herbal practitioner has a number of remedies which can be used for childhood ailments such as measles, mumps, chickenpox, etc., and can be consulted for these.

Circulation

Often due to heart problems, poor circulation is also commonly associated with the degeneration of blood vessels, the hardening or weakening of the tiny muscle fibres in the vessel walls. Faulty diet can increase blood viscosity, which leads to sluggish circulation in the smallest blood vessels, the capillaries. Nervous control of artery walls can cause increased contraction, inhibiting the blood supply, and faults in the fluid balance of the body can allow fluid to remain in body tissues, which also slows down the circulation. The herbal practitioner has a number of remedies which he will prescribe for his patients according to his findings on examination. Experienced practitioners have prepared formulae from their own experience in practice which can benefit circulatory problems. Such are Napier's Cayenne tablets and Roberts' 'Drops of Life' mixture, which could be supplemented by rutin tablets, buckwheat tea, and a diet which includes wheat germ, sunflower seeds, watercress and plenty of fresh salads. Salt should be avoided.

Coeliac Disease

This condition should be under the care of a practitioner. It is a disease which can affect both children and adults, in which the body has no ability to absorb gluten (the protein content of wheat and other grains) and fats. The cause is not known, though an hereditary factor has been found in some cases. A gluten-free diet is essential, and a few children have been found to be sensitive to cow's milk. Herbs which improve liver function, digestion and assimilation will be used by the herbal practitioner, together with remedies to relieve flatulence and abdominal discomfort.

Colic

Acute, often intense, pain which fluctuates according to the muscular action of the bowel (peristalsis), can be due to gases in the bowels formed from the fermentation of badly-digested foods, usually carbohydrates. A hot infusion of peppermint, avens or catmint (one teaspoonful of any one to a teacupful of boiling water, with a pinch of powdered ginger added) will give quick relief. Antispas is also useful, a teaspoonful in half a teacup of hot water, sweetened very slightly, sipped whilst hot. Wild yam is also a useful herb for pain in the abdomen. One experienced herbal practitioner, Frank Roberts, had much success with his Nervous Dyspepsia tablets taken with a hot infusion of his 'Drops of Life'.

If colic occurs frequently it would be wise to consult a practitioner to ascertain the cause.

Colitis

Inflammation of the colon can arise as the result of some infection in the gastro-intestinal system, or some longstanding irritation to the lining of the colon, for example the use of strong purgatives. It is most commonly found in self-conscious, shy individuals, and seldom starts after the age of thirty. Mucus colitis is the milder form, in which there is frequent bowel action with quantities of mucus in the stool and colicky pain in the abdomen. Slippery elm should be taken at least three times daily and also a cupful of agrimony infusion. Add one teaspoonful of agrimony herb to a teacupful of boiling water, cover and leave to cool. Strain and add one teaspoonful of composition essence. This should be taken up to three times daily. A useful combination of herbs for mucus colitis which can also be beneficial for the ulcerative form is equal quantities of cranesbill, agrimony and marshmallow root powdered.

Add 1oz (25g) of the mixture to 1pint (0.5 litre) of boiling water, cover and leave to cool. A pinch of caraway seeds or aniseed chewed after meals will help prevent flatulence.

Ulcerative colitis can develop from untreated or unresolved mucus colitis. Diarrhoea is almost constant, blood and mucus are passed, and there is frequent discomfort in the abdomen. Add comfrey root to the agrimony, cranesbill and marshmallow recipe given above, slicing or chopping it finely before including it. Roberts' Golden Seal tablets and Gerard Fenulin tablets have proved to be of great help in this condition.

Colitis is considered by many authorities to be a psychosomatic condition and so nervines such as skull cap, valerian and chamomile flowers would be useful taken either in tablet form or as herbal tea. Naturopathic psychotherapy or counselling could be a great help.

Natural yogurt with a little honey added should be eaten daily to improve the condition within the colon.

Diet may have to be bland initially, the range of high fibre foods being introduced gradually as improvement takes place.

Common Colds and Chills

When the first feeling of chilliness, cold feet, sore throat or sneezing indicates a cold is developing take hot infusions of any herb given below, go straight to bed with a flask of the hot infusion and a flask of lemon juice and honey in hot water. Take the drinks frequently (every half-hour is not too often), avoid food and stay in bed until perspiration has taken place and the temperature is back to normal.

- Peppermint, angelica herb and balm, in equal quantities

- Elderflower and peppermint

- Yarrow, hyssop and horehound (for a cold on the chest)

- Sage (if the throat is sore) one teaspoonful to ½ pint (0.25 litre) boiling, water, cover closely

- Elderflowers and lime blossom in equal quantities, in the early stages if much sneezing occurs

- Composition essence, one or two teaspoonfuls to a teacup of hot water, for chilliness

- Take plenty of vitamin C, at least a 200mg tablet every hour between the herbal teas.

The herbs are to be prepared as normal infusions and taken in wineglassful doses. Potter's or Napier's Composition Essence or Abbott's Sure Cure are good bottled remedies, also Potter's EPC mixture. Following the advice given above, avoiding food and having only fruit juices and then fresh fruit when the appetite has returned will quickly clear the cold and prevent any long aftermath of catarrh.

Conjunctivitis

The first remedy to spring to the mind for any eye problems is eyebright. A few drops of the tincture to an eyebath of pure water, used two or three times each day will help relieve this painful complaint. An infusion of elderflowers, 1 oz (25g) simmered for five minutes in 1 pint (0.5 litre) of water, left to infuse for ten minutes then filtered through a paper coffee filter will be found to be soothing. So will

German chamomile flowers, prepared by adding 1 oz (25g) to 1 pint (0.5 litre) of cold water, covered by a well fitting lid and brought to the boil. Remove immediately from the heat, leave to infuse for twenty minutes without removing the lid, then filter. Use either of these, undiluted, in the eyebath and also soak pads of cotton wool to apply as compresses over the eyes. A few drops of tincture of myrrh may be added to the whole infusion, for its antiseptic properties.

Use bottled spring water for bathing the eyes; use an eye bathful for one eye at a time.

Constipation

Constipation means different things to different people: for the purpose of discussing remedies it is enough to consider a state in which there is less than a daily bowel action. Causes of constipation should be sought and corrected whenever possible. The most common reason for constipation is lack of dietary fibre, due to a diet which consists almost totally of refined and 'convenience' foods.

The diet should be changed but remedies to take in the meantime are:

- Senna pods - take five or more, tear or crush them, add a pinch of powdered ginger and a cupful of boiling water, cover and leave to stand overnight. Drink the strained liquid before breakfast

- Cascara - most easily taken in the form of liquid extract, which is obtainable from chemists. The dose of this can be varied as required - start with a small dose of, say, five drops in a little water at bedtime, increasing it as required

- Linseed - a tablespoonful of the seeds may be soaked in water overnight, then added to breakfast cereal to add bulk to the diet

- Liquorice root - a pleasant-tasting gentle laxative, which can be taken alone or added to either senna or cascara to improve the flavour. Peel the sticks before use, add 2 oz (50g) to 2 pints (1 litre) of cold water. Bring to the boil and simmer very gently for ten minutes. Stand until cool, then strain. Take a wineglassful three or more times daily, or add a wineglassful to the dose of either senna or cascara.

Improve the diet by having a wholegrain cereal or porridge at breakfast, instead of the soft pulpy refined cereals. Eat wholewheat bread, increase the amount of salads and vegetables in the diet. Stewed prunes or figs should be taken each day. There are, of course, a number of proprietary herbal laxatives available.

Convalescence

A number of herbs may be taken, either alone or in combination, to assist the body to recoup strength during this stage of an illness. Afine remedy is vervain, especially when depression seems to hinder recovery. A wineglassful of the normal infusion three or four times daily will bring about cheerfulness and general improvement. Balm tea will also help by soothing the nerves and improving appetite.

A wineglassful several times daily, with a slice of lemon and a little honey added, will soon have a tonic effect. A gruel of oats is a fine remedy for nervous exhaustion, and will have a good tonic effect on heart muscle. Boil l oz (25g) of medium oatmeal in 3 pints (1.5 litres) of water until reduced to 2 pints (1 litre). Add a teaspoonful of molasses and a little honey. Take a cupful several times daily. If taken at bedtime it will help to induce sleep. A superb herbal tonic, helping to improve the appetite, is a combination of equal quantities of balmony herb, finely chopped gentian root, poplar bark and peruvian bark, also chopped finely, simmered gently for fifteen minutes, having added 1oz (25g) of the mixture to 1 1/2 pints (0.75 litre) of water. No sweetening should be added to this; a wineglassful should be taken three times daily before meals.

Corns

Some herbal practitioners have their own preparations for corns, Roberts' Corn and Callous ointment, for example, or Potter's Walk Easy ointment, which is obtainable from health food stores.

A leaf from the houseleek plant, a small succulent plant which grows on old roofs and old walls, if applied fresh to a corn, bound in place and renewed night and morning, will soften a corn. Lemon juice applied has also been found effective.

Keep the feet in good condition and wear well-fitting shoes.

Coronary Thrombosis

A coronary thrombosis needs swift professional attention to save the life of the patient. Prevention of the condition and its recurrence depends on diet, the life-style and temperament of the patient, and on persistence in taking the right herbal remedies over a long period of time.

Yarrow herb has anti-thrombotic properties, a wineglassful of cold infusion could judiciously be taken twice daily. To strengthen the heart and circulatory system and to improve the quality of blood, a tea of hawthorn flowers and leaves, yarrow and melilot should be taken three times daily. Prepare by taking 1oz (25g) of the mixed herbs, add to 1 pint (0.5 litre) of boiling water, cover and leave to stand for ten minutes. The dose is a wineglassful. It would also be useful to take hawthorn and rutin tablets, which are readily available.

Animal fats should be eliminated completely from the diet. Asemi-vegetarian diet would be preferable and large meals should be avoided, Biosalt should replace table salt, and dandelion coffee and Luaka or Mate tea should be taken instead of ordinary tea and coffee. There is often a lack of silica and potash, and to replenish the body's supplies one or two teaspoonsful of molasses should be taken each day. It would be wise to consult a herbal practitioner for treatment of this condition.

See also Arteriosclerosis.

Coughs

A cough should not be suppressed, as it is a symptom revealing either inflammation of the mucous membrane lining the air passages or an attempt to clear mucus from the lungs. Herbal expectorants will aid the removal of mucus: prepare a mixture of equal quantities of hyssop, comfrey root (finely sliced), white horehound, coltsfoot and liquorice sticks (peeled and chopped). Take about 2 ½ oz (60g), add to 2 pints (1 litre) cold water, bring to the boil and simmer gently for fifteen minutes. Strain through a fine cloth or paper coffee filter. Take a wineglassful three or four times daily, having a few sips when required to relieve a fit of coughing.

If the cough is a dry one, take 1oz (25g) each of peeled and chopped liquorice sticks and marshmallow root, simmer gently in 2 pints (1 litre) of water for fifteen minutes, then add a teaspoonful of thyme and a good pinch of crushed caraway seeds. Replace the lid and leave until cool. Take a wineglassful four times daily. Elecampane root is another good cough remedy, helping to expel mucus, and having slight antibiotic properties. Oil of eucalyptus, inhaled, will help clear the air passages.

Mention has been made of only a few remedies which the herbal practitioner will use in the treatment of coughs.

Many more are available; some of them in the prepared mixtures such as Heath & Heather's cough mixture,

Napier's chest and cough tablets, and others. Milk and dairy products should be avoided until the cough and any catarrh have cleared completely.

Cramp

This painful spasm in muscles can be due to circulatory problems or to certain deficiencies of minerals or vitamins. Imbalance of salt in the body, either too much or too little can lead to cramp; therefore an experiment must be made in decreasing or increasing the amount taken. There may be a calcium deficiency, so take one calcium tablet daily with food. Calcium lactate is most easily absorbed by the body. One stalwart herbalist, Albert Orb ell, recommends a mustard foot-bath to be taken up to three times per week.

Add one tablespoonful of mustard to enough hot water to cover the feet and ankles, bathe the feet for three minutes, splashing the calves. Dry carefully, and rub well in an upward direction with a good herbal liniment. In addition, at bedtime, take a wineglassful of a mixture made from one teaspoonful each of cloves, lemon juice and honey in 1/2 pint (0.25 litre) of boiling water covered and allowed to stand for twenty-four hours, with a tablespoonful of ginger wine added. Further remedies are vitamin E, starting with 100m daily, or vitamin B6.

Croup

This unpleasant barking cough with hoarseness is commonly experienced by young children. It may be the aftermath of a cold and cough or due to some new infection or allergy. Add one teaspoonful each of vervain and coltsfoot herb to a teacupful of boiling water, cover and allow to stand for ten minutes. Strain through a paper coffee filter to prevent the fine down from the leaves irritating the throat. Heat again, adding some honey, and drink it hot three times daily. The dose is a teaspoonful for an infant, increasing to a tablespoonful for a five-year-old. A teaspoonful of garlic-infused honey (see Bronchitis, page 36) in a teacupful of hot water could be given to a small child, but not to an infant. Rub the chest and throat with Olbas oil, and stop all dairy products until the condition has cleared.

Cystitis

Inflammation of the bladder is becoming more common, due in part to use of the contraceptive pill or antibiotics, to lack of personal hygiene, in some cases to gonococcal infection and to lowered level of general health.

A number of herbs are used to relieve the acute inflammation and burning. A good combination is equal quantities of marshmallow leaves, uva ursi, sage and horsetail, mixed well together. One tablespoonful is added to a large cupful of boiling water, simmered gently for five minutes and allowed to cool (still covered). This should be taken two or three times daily. Other useful remedies are buchu leaves, couch grass, cranesbill, meadowsweet and burdock root. They may be taken alone or combined, prepared as above. Pellitory of the wall has been found helpful, especially when there is a painful feeling as if the bladder is distended. A teaspoonful of the herb to a teacupful of boiling water covered and allowed to cool, should be taken twice or three times daily.

Some excellent tablets and preparations for cystitis are available from health food stores, Potter's Antitis tablets for example, or Roberts' uva ursi tablets or Gerard cystitis tablets. Drink plenty of barley water to supplement the medication. An excellent recipe is given by Juliette de

Bairacli Levy in her *Illustrated Herbal Handbook:* you will need 4 oz (115g) whole barley, 2 oz (55g) honey, peel of half a small lemon (well washed) and 1 pint of water. First boil the barley in a little water and drain off the water.

Then pour a pint of water over the cleaned barley, and add the lemon peel. Simmer gently until the barley is soft.

Remove from heat, allow to steep and add the honey when the barley water is 'new milk' warm. (There are many ways of making barley water: this is an old-fashioned recipe and a good-tasting one.)

Avoid acid-forming foods such as tomatoes, spinach, vinegar and pickles, rhubarb and gooseberries. An herbal practitioner would help to overcome cystitis if the condition persists in spite of the measures recommended above.

Cysts

As welling or sac filled with liquid or semi-liquid substance may arise as the result of blockage in the outlet of some gland or body cavity. A cyst should be dealt with by a practitioner.

Dandruff

As with skin disorders and the condition of the hair, dandruff is related to general health. Therefore follow appropriate measures in addition to dealing directly with the dandruff itself.

An infusion of nettles (leaves, tops and stems) taken in wineglassful doses three times daily will provide the body with minerals to improve the scalp; massage the scalp every day with a lotion made from nettle seeds to stimulate the circulation. Cut the tops from seeding nettles and, wearing gloves, shake the tops over a large sheet of paper to collect the seeds. It will probably be necessary to include some of the flowering tops in the infusion. Make a normal infusion, straining off a little each time it is required. Take also a teacupful of clivers tea each day. This herb is rich in silica and is good for hair, teeth and nails.

Deafness

There is no magic remedy for deafness. If it is due to catarrh a diligent course of treatment for that condition could bring about improvement. If the deafness is due to nerve disorder - not nerve damage - follow the advice given under the heading

Nervous Disorders (page 105). Slight deafness might, in some cases, be helped by improved nutrition to the nervous system.

Debility

Debility, or lack of strength, is the natural sequel of prolonged illness, stress, anxiety or faulty diet, coupled with a deficiency of B vitamins and minerals.

The first step to take is to change the diet to incorporate whole grains and at least fifty per cent of daily food as raw salads, vegetables and fruits. These foods contain essential minerals and trace elements which produce chemical stimuli to create energy (see *Handbook of Health* by

Constance Mellor). Include nuts, seeds, some mixed proteins, and avoid stimulants such as coffee, alcohol, tobacco, vinegar and strong tea.

Combine 1oz (25g) each of agrimony, avens, chamomile flowers, poplar bark and gentian root (finely chopped), mix well and simmer 1 oz (25g) of the mixture very gently in 2 pints (1 litre) of water for ten minutes. Allow to cool, then strain and take a wineglassful before meals. Gentian root alone, prepared as above, acts as a good tonic for the liver, appetite or digestive system. The taste is bitter, so add a little mint, basil or sweet cicely, but not honey, and take a dessertspoonful before meals. A number of other remedies are prescribed by the herbal practitioner according to the patient's individual needs, including a weak infusion of tansy herb taken in small doses, agnus castus, ginseng and lucerne.

It is necessary to have adequate rest, a walk in the fresh air each day, breathing deeply whilst doing so, and a positive mental attitude. If energy and vitality are not restored by the measures advised, a practitioner should be consulted to find and deal with the underlying cause.

Depression

There is no need for depression to commit one to life-long dependence on tranquillizers or anti-depressant drugs. A wide range of herbs is available to the herbal practitioner, who makes an assessment of the patient's general health problems when treating depression.

The condition usually arises when the body is in a state of poor nutrition and vitality is low, for example after childbirth, severe illness, even after influenza, or prolonged stress. It is also in some cases due to an allergic reaction to some item in the diet, even - rarely - to drinking-water.

The ever-useful antispasmodic tincture is a good base from which to start treatment, a teaspoonful in half a teacupful of warm sweetened water taken two or three times daily, or when feeling particularly low. Between the doses of antispas a wineglassful of vervain will improve digestion, help regain strength and counteract the nervy, depressed feelings. Lavender tea is useful too, being a good nerve tonic; add three or four flowering spikes to a cupful of boiling water with a little honey (lavender honey if possible), cover closely and drink the strained liquid when cool. An infusion of borage leaves, normal infusion, in wineglassful doses night and morning will give rise to cheerful feelings, as will chervil.

Ginseng, as a general tonic which influences all the systems of the body, can be used to help overcome depression. If the powdered root is available, mix 3 oz (75g) to a smooth paste with 1 oz (25g) of honey. Keep in a screw-top jar and take one teaspoonful of this in a cupful of boiling water twice daily before meals. Leave it to stand for ten minutes before drinking.

Follow a good diet. If preparation of nutritious meals is too much trouble, as it so often is during depression, take three brewer's yeast tablets three times daily with food, make sure that a good wholemeal bread replaces white bread, and have the simplest meals, providing they consist of really good wholesome ingredients.

Consult an herbal practitioner, whose treatment will help a great deal toward bringing back the zest for life.

Dermatitis

This inflammation of the skin can arise on the hands as a result of contact with harsh detergents or some other irritant, or it can be due to low grade health and a diet deficient in vitamins A, B complex, and vegetable oils.

The herbal remedies described under Skin Problems will be of help, especially echinacea and blue flag root. Chickweed ointment, or slippery elm and marshmallow cream should be applied during the day and at bedtime. The diet should consist of lots of salads, green vegetables, raw carrots, and a dessertspoonful of sunflower seed oil daily. Two B complex tablets with meals twice daily and 2,500IU of vitamin A should supplement the diet.

Commonsense practicalities, such as the wearing of gloves (cotton ones inside rubber ones may be necessary) when using any form of detergent, and the limited use of a gentle soap will contribute to improving the skin.

Consult an herbal practitioner if the condition fails to clear.

Diarrhoea

Acute diarrhoea occurs when the body is trying to rid itself of some infection, toxin or unwanted food substance.

Food poisoning, whether mild or severe causes vomiting and diarrhoea for twenty-four to forty-eight hours, and should be helped by drinking plenty of warm water with a little antispas added. Composition essence is useful too, as it is anti-bacterial in its action. The condition should be allowed to run its course, but if it continues beyond two or three days the cause should be sought.

A more persistent diarrhoea can be dealt with by astringent remedies such as agrimony, plantain leaves, tormentil, bistort or geranium. An infusion of any of these, prepared as a normal infusion with a pinch of powdered ginger, cinnamon or crushed caraway seeds added to the infusion whilst cooling, will help. Wineglassful doses taken three or four times daily should be adequate. An infusion of blackberry leaves is beneficial too, dose and method as above. Garlic oil capsules should be taken each night, and the occasional teaspoonful dose of composition essence in hot water will help.

Spells of diarrhoea alternating with constipation, or any prolonged change from normal bowel action without an associated change in diet, must be referred to a practitioner for diagnosis and treatment.

See also Colitis.

Digestive Disorders

The herbal practitioner has a cornucopia of remedies to deal with the varied problems which arise in the digestive system, from anise seeds to avert flatulence to zingiber (ginger) to ease abdominal pains, and which will, on occasion, prevent travel-sickness. Persistent and recurrent digestive symptoms which do not respond to any remedies or respond only briefly, must be investigated thoroughly.

Simple indigestion, which can be due to a slight disturbance in the liver function, will often be eased quite quickly by an infusion of centaury herb taken three times daily in half-teacupful doses between meals. The same herb, when combined with an equal quantity of angelica herb, will improve catarrh of the stomach. Dairy products must be eliminated from the diet to help the herbs clear the catarrh. Dandelion root is a good stimulus to digestion, acting as it does on the liver, pancreas and intestines. A few of the young leaves included in the daily salad will be sufficient in mild cases of indigestion.

Dyspepsia responds to balm tea or to peppermint tea: a wineglassful taken a short time after each meal daily will have the required effect. Pains in the stomach will often be eased quickly by chewing a pinch of coriander seeds, or averted by having them just before meals. A teaspoonful of antispasmodic tincture in hot water will also ease stomach pains due to wind or muscular spasm.

All of the culinary herbs - caraway, fennel, marjoram, bay leaves, thyme, rosemary and others - will aid digestion when included in meals. Nervous dyspepsia is eased by a wineglassful of chamomile tea, catmint (taken cold) or rosemary taken before meals. A teaspoonful of anyone of these added to a teacupful of boiling water, covered and left to cool, strained off as required, will be adequate.

Slippery elm should be taken regularly for its soothing properties. Mix a teaspoonful of the powdered bark to a smooth paste with a little honey; gradually add a cupful of boiling water or milk and water. Take this two or three times daily, according to the severity of the digestive problems. It may be wise to have a short course of remedies for the nervous system to reinforce the action of the digestives. Follow a simple diet, eating only when relaxed, chewing food well and drinking between meals.

See also Acidity, Appetite, Flatulence,, Gastric Ulcer , Gastritis.

Diverticulitis

Small pockets or pouches form in the walls of the colon, sometimes occurring naturally and being of no consequence.

Inflammation of these diverticuli causes pain and some discomfort on either side of the abdomen. Bowel action is irregular, constipation usually heralding an attack.

Slippery elm taken at least twice daily will be soothing to the lining of the colon, alternated with either peppermint tea to relieve pain and reduce fermentation, or a cupful of chamomile tea taken before meals. Prepare the chamomile by adding a tablespoonful of the flowers to a large teacupful of boiling water, cover and leave to stand for fifteen minutes. Strain when required, and add a few drops of lemon juice to reinforce its antiseptic action.

Follow a whole food diet but not one which is *excessive* in fibre, i.e. eat whole-wheat bread if it can be tolerated, but avoid a coarse bran or muesli at breakfast. Losing weight, if overweight, will help to overcome diverticulitis.

Take linseed each day, one cupful first thing in the morning, more later in the day between meals if necessary. Allow 1 oz

(25g) of crushed linseed to stand overnight in 2 pints (1 litre) of pure cold water. Linseed is demulcent, and is soothing and healing to all parts of the digestive tract.

The dose must be adjusted to individual requirements as large doses can be laxative. The seeds are often added to the diet to add bulk in cases of obstinate constipation.

Lemon or liquorice may be added to vary the flavour.

Diverticulitis may need persistence with treatment, and advice from a herbal practitioner will be reassuring.

Dizziness

This unpleasant sensation can be due to a number of problems: a temporary virus infection in the ears, abnormal blood-pressure, anxiety, exhaustion, anaemia, or liver problems. It is necessary to find the cause before any treatment can be considered. Balm is a good remedy if the dizziness is due to anxiety and nervous problems. A normal infusion taken in wineglassful doses two or three times daily is generally adequate.

Dropsy

Dropsy, an abnormal accumulation of fluid in the body, is a symptom of an underlying condition which must be treated professionally. General health must be built up and the function of the liver and kidneys, often a contributory cause, must be improved in order to remove toxins and impurities from the system. Herbal teas and dietary measures can be used in conjunction with treatment if necessary. Combine 1oz (25g) each of broom tops and agrimony with ½ oz (12.5g) each of juniper berries and lily of the valley, simmer gently for fifteen minutes in 2 pints (1 litre) of water. Cool, strain and take one wineglassful three or four times daily.

Another useful formula is equal quantities of broom tops, agrimony and dandelion root. Simmer 1 oz (25g) of the mixture gently for fifteen minutes, and take four times daily in wineglassful doses.

A salt-free diet, which includes plenty of celery, parsley, asparagus and green leafy vegetables, with strict avoidance of coffee, will support the herbal teas. A number of proprietary remedies are available. Roberts' Black Willow

Compound tablets, Gerard's or Heath & Heather's Buchu tablets and others, will be found useful, but it must be stressed that this condition should have professional diagnosis and treatment. The cause of the dropsy must be treated.

Duodenal Ulcer

An excessive flow of stomach digestive acid, hydrochloric acid, irritates the wall of the duodenum and eventually forms an ulcer. The patient may often suffer years of 'indigestion', biliousness, and general discomfort after eating fatty foods, and much heartburn, before this condition arises.

The first herbal remedy to be taken is meadowsweet, an alkaline herb which will neutralize the acid to start the healing process. Comfrey leaf tea and marshmallow root, taken in wineglassful doses two or three times daily, will soothe and help to heal the mucous membrane lining of the duodenum. Herbal teas should be taken at body temperature, not cold. A cupful of slippery elm should be taken three times daily, made by mixing a teaspoonful of the powder to a paste with a little honey, and gradually adding a cupful of hot water or milk and water. A little nutmeg may be grated on top to aid digestion and to add a different flavour.

The diet must be amended to exclude fried foods, refined carbohydrates, vinegar, spices and pickles. Food should be chewed well.

See also Gastric Ulcer.

Dysentery

One of the most simple and effective remedies for dysentery (inflammation of the bowel), is agrimony. A wineglassful taken cold three or four times daily will help ease the pain and will control looseness and frequent straining. Its astringent properties will also help controlany blood and mucus, especially if it is combined with an equal quantity of plantain leaves. A good remedy to use if blood appears in the motion is comfrey root, 1oz (25g) of the finely chopped root is added to 2 pints (1 litre) of cold water, brought up to the boil, and simmered gently to reduce the liquid by one quarter. A wineglassful can be taken as frequently as needed, up to two-hourly intervals throughout the day. Amore powerful astringent is bistort.

Take about six inches of the root, chop finely, add to ½ pint (0.25 litres) of boiling water, and simmer gently for five minutes. Take two tablespoonfuls before meals.

A remedy which should be freely available in spring and summer is fresh blackberry leaves. A handful simmered gently for five minutes in 2 pints (1 litre) of boiling water and allowed to cool, can be taken in teacupful doses three or more times daily. Marshmallow is soothing, and can be taken between the more astringent remedies to ease the inflammation. Add 1 oz

(25g) of the leaves to 2 pints (1 litre) of cold water, stand for ten minutes then bring to the boil.

Remove immediately from heat, keeping covered, and leave to infuse for a further ten minutes. Honey may be added at this stage if desired. Strain, and take a teacupful three times daily.

In addition to any of the above remedies, take three garlic oil capsules at bedtime.

Dyspepsia

A feeling of, indigestion' and fullness after meals can often be relieved by wild yam, peppermint tea or balm tea taken immediately after a meal. Food should be chewed thoroughly, and drinks should only be taken between meals. Potter's Indigestion mixture and Heath & Heather's

Indigestion tablets would both be helpful, Napier's

Indigestion tablets also give relief. If the condition does not clear up the help of a practitioner should be sought.

Ear Disorders

Children frequently suffer from earache when catarrhal infection extends to the Eustachian tube. Both earache and infection should be treated as catarrh. A little warmed almond oil can be dropped into the ear, or antispasmodic tincture massaged gently around the ear and a few drops, warmed, applied on cotton wool in the ear. An infusion of yarrow herb can be applied on cotton wool as a hot compress outside the ear, and a few drops, just warm, applied in the ear on cotton wool. Hyssop herb infusion can be used in exactly the same way. Melilot infusion, taken three times daily will help to ease the earache.

Wax in the ears can be softened by applying a few drops of almond oil each night. Apply it in one ear at a time, lying with that ear uppermost. Do not put dry cotton wool in the ear as it will soak up the oil; moisten a small plug of cotton wool in warm water, squeeze it almost dry then apply a drop or two of the oil before inserting it in the ear. Do not drop oil or lotion into the ear if the drum has been damaged, apply the medication on cotton wool.

For noises in the ears, see Tinnitus.

Eczema

Eczema is a symptom rather than an actual disease, and may be the temporary reaction to some food item or drug.

A common allergen is cow's milk, and changing to goat's milk will often bring about a cure of infantile or childhood eczema. There may also be a background of 'nerves' or anxiety which must be dealt with. Individual treatment is necessary, but a good combination of herbs is equal quantities of yellow dock root, clivers, blue flag root, wild carrot and fumitory. Mix them well, add 2 oz *(50g)* to 2 pints (1 litre) of cold water, bring to the boil and simmer gently for fifteen minutes. Remove from heat, strain when cool and take a wineglassful after meals. (For details of children's' doses see Children's Ailments). Dry eczema, with dry skin all over, will often benefit from the inclusion of one to three tablespoonfuls of sunflower seed oil in the diet, and plenty of watercress. Indeed, watercress has been used successfully as a poultice on eczema. It should be boiled in enough water to cover until it is a soft mass, then mixed with fine oatmeal and applied in muslin as a poultice.

Change every twenty-four hours.

A soothing lotion can be made from plantain leaves, infusing 1 oz *(25g)* in 1 pint *(0.5* litre) of boiling water for ten minutes. The strained liquid is used as a lotion; apply freely to relieve itching. The leaves may be applied as a poultice to particularly bad patches if desired. Weleda Sambucus compound is also used as a soothing lotion or compress. A number of other remedies are used by the herbal practitioner either as internal medicine or as lotion.

Each case needs individual treatment.

Emphysema

This condition is a chronic distension of the air-sacs in the lungs, in which air is retained and cannot be exhaled. It is due to repeated, prolonged coughing, is a sequel to chronic bronchitis or is due to many years in an occupation which demanded hard breathing such as blowing wind instruments or lifting heavy objects. .

Equal quantities of comfrey root combined with liquorice root, simmered for fifteen minutes, 1oz *(25g)* of the mixture to 1pint *(0.5* litre) of water with a pinch of crushed anise seeds added when it is cooling, can help. The dose is a wineglassful three or four times daily. In addition, the measures advised for chronic bronchitis (page 36) will probably give some relief. Daily breathing exercises which consist of trying to breathe *out* as long as possible, relaxing the body at the same time, are important.

Enteritis

Inflammation of the small intestine can be treated in the same way as dysentery and gastro-enteritis, by fasting until the symptoms have abated, by drinking herbal teas freely and by drinking slippery elm several times each day.

A combination of 1oz *(25g)* each of oak bark, barberry bark, agrimony and raspberry leaves is useful, added as 1 oz *(25g)* of the mixed herbs to 1 1/2 pints (0.75 litre) cold water, brought to boiling point and simmered very gently for fifteen minutes. The dose is up to a teacupful every three hours in severe cases. Marshmallow tea could be taken in between the doses, as could a decoction of cornfrey root.

Two garlic capsules taken at bedtime will be a useful antibiotic.

Enuresis

There is seldom a structural or pathological reason for persistent bed-wetting, but a check-up by a practitioner would confirm this. The cause is almost always emotional or psychological, and may occur when a new baby arrives in the family, or when changes at school make the child feel insecure or insignificant. The child should be given plenty of love and reassurance, and the reason for its anxiety should be sought. A wholesome diet which contains plenty of green leafy vegetables, sunflower seeds and very little refined sugar is advisable. Drinks during the evening should be avoided and so should too much excitement before bedtime.

A tea prepared from horse tail herb is often very successful: ½ oz (12.5g) to 1 ½ pints (0.75 litre) water, simmered gently for fifteen minutes, strained when cool.

The dose is one tablespoonful two or three times daily for a child seven to eight years old, a dessertspoonful for a younger child. Corn silk is also effective, half a tablespoonful added to a cupful of boiling water, and simmered very gently for ten minutes, adding molasses to flavour.

Give two teaspoonfuls twice daily to a child of five or six. St John's Wort herb can be prepared in the same way, two teaspoonfuls given at bedtime.

Epilepsy

Not a condition for self-treatment. However, care of general health, together with some harmless tisanes, will be found to make some improvement.

Herbal remedies which have been found useful in this condition and which could be taken regularly in conjunction with other medication include mistletoe, valerian and hyssop. Anyone of these can be taken at one time. Hyssop is prepared as a normal infusion, two tablespoonfuls being taken before meals. Add 1/2oz (12.5g) of chopped valerian root to 1 pint (0.5 litre) of cold water, heat slowly and gently to almost boiling point, remove immediately from heat and leave to cool. Honey and a trace of peppermint may be added to disguise the flavour. Take two tablespoonfuls before meals. If using mistletoe, chop 1oz (25g) of the twigs and leaves, add to 1pint (0.5 litres) of cold water, cover and leave to soak all night. Do not heat and do not *use* the berries. The dose is a wineglassful before meals.

To make some improvement in general vitality have adequate rest, don't get over-tired and take some gentle exercise in the fresh air, doing deep breathing to provide the body and the brain with plenty of oxygen. Vitamin B complex would be a useful dietary supplement. The measures advised are not claimed to cure epilepsy, but to benefit the general health.

Erysipelas

When available fresh, apply newly gathered, washed chickweed over the erysipelas sores, cover with a washed lettuce leaf and bind gently in place. Renew every three hours. Alternatively, plantain leaves, pulped and mixed with a little hot water, should be spread on clean cotton or linen cloth, bound into place and changed every twelve hours.

Almost specifically used for erysipelas, the root of golden seal is an expensive remedy. It has soothing healing properties. If the powdered root is available, steep half a teaspoonful in a teacupful of near-boiling water for ten minutes and apply as a poultice. Echinacea tablets or tea should be taken, together with good diuretics such as divers, dandelion, and buchu, adding blue flag root and red dover flowers. Avoid food, taking plenty of pure water and diluted fruit juices.

Eye Problems

It has been said that 'The eyes are the windows of the soul'. To the practitioner they are often the means of seeing the patient's health; the state of the white indicates much concerning the blood vessels and liver, the tissues around the eyes can reveal kidney disorders, and the retina reveals much else. Any persistent or chronic eye problem must not be dealt with by home treatment; professional advice must be sought.

For tired, aching eyes a number of easily available herbs can be used to bathe the eyes and to apply as compresses. Eyebright herb is first and foremost, or elderflower, fennel seed, or raspberry leaves. To prepare any of these, add one teaspoonful of the selected herb to a teacupful of boiling water (using bottled spring water). Cover and leave to cool.

Strain through a paper coffee filter and use the liquid as an eyebath, bathing one eye a few times then discarding the liquid. If the eyes are at all inflamed or infected, always use fresh lotion for each eye. The lotion can also be used to soak pads of cotton wool or lint for compresses.

Sore eyes are relieved by a chickweed lotion. Wash a handful of fresh chickweed, cover it with boiling water and leave to cool. Strain through fine cloth and use the liquid to make a compress. Styes on the eye are relieved by compresses of elderflowers, marigold flowers or nasturtium seeds. The seeds should be crushed, covered in boiling water and the whole applied as a compress on lint. Styes are a sign of lowered vitality and impurities in the bloodstream, and treatment to the eyes should be supplemented by tonics and blood purifiers. (See Blood Disorders).

Chamomile flowers make a soothing eye bath, and 1oz (25g) added to ½ pint (0.25 litre) of boiling water, allowed to infuse for ten minutes then strained through a paper coffee filter, will relax and ease tired eyes. The flowers can be used as a compress, leaving in place for an hour.

Fainting

A tendency to fainting may be due to nervousness or to poor circulation inhibiting circulation to the brain. One of the finest remedies to take is rosemary, as its stimulating and tonic properties will both improve the circulation and strengthen the nerves. A teaspoonful of the herb to a teacupful of boiling water, covered and allowed to cool, should be taken, warm, half a cupful in the morning and half at bedtime. St John's Wort is an astringent and antidepressant which can be very effective when there is occasional fainting. A wineglassful of the normal infusion three times daily will, in most cases, correct the condition.

Peppermint tea is also beneficial, taken two or three times each day. Roberts' Valerian compound tablets and Nerfood tablets have also been successful.

If no improvement takes place after persisting with these remedies, seek the advice of a practitioner.

Feet

Distortion of the shape of the feet due to fashionable pointed-toe shoes, and strain on ankle, leg and pelvic muscles by high thin heels can cause more misery in later life than can be realized. Massage and manipulation by an osteopath will often help, and exercises will be of benefit too.

Footbaths can be used to give relief to aching feet: equal quantities of nettles and marshmallow leaves, 1oz (25g) of each to 2 pints (1 litre) of boiling water, allowed to cool to body temperature and strained into a bowl large enough to stand the feet in, with enough warm water added to cover feet and come up to the ankles. Bathe the feet for ten minutes, sponge with cool water and dry thoroughly.

For perspiring feet a daily footbath containing a 1 oz (25g) infusion of horse tail, plus a salt spoonful of sea salt, bathed for ten minutes, reinforced by a wineglassful of diuretic infusion three times daily will correct excessive perspiration.

Lovage herb is a deodorant and can also be used for this condition, 'a handful of fresh leaves infused for ten minutes then added to a footbath.

The exercises described under the heading, Varicose Veins, will be of benefit to the feet, and should be carried out daily.

Fevers

A raised temperature with signs of feverishness is a sign that the body is endeavouring to throw off toxic wastes, and should be assisted by herbal teas to promote perspiration.

Infusions of hot yarrow, elderflower and peppermint, boneset herb, sage, clivers or meadowsweet herb, given in wineglassful doses every hour or so should be continued until a good perspiration takes place, at which time sleep often completes the first stage. The body can be sponged quickly with a cloth or towel wrung out in cold water, taking care that the sufferer does not get chilled. The patient should stay in bed until the temperature is normal, and should have only diluted lemon and other fruit juices in addition to the herbal teas - no food at all.

Any of the herbal remedies can be given as cool drinks when the body is back to normal: clivers if there is backache, peppermint for nausea or headaches, boneset if the limbs are aching. Verbena tea can be taken at this time to aid recovery. See also Convalescence, page 48. Do not waste any time trying herbal teas or any other methods in sudden very high temperatures in children; call a practitioner immediately.

Fibrositis
An over-worked term meaning inflammation of the white fibrous body tissue, especially that which provides a thin covering of muscle. Rub well with good herbal liniment - Olbas oil, Weleda massage balm or some other, and take a wineglassful three times daily of the following: add 1 oz (25g) each of meadowsweet, nettle, yarrow, yellow dock root and bogbean, to 2 pints (1 litre) of boiling water, and simmer very gently in a covered pan for fifteen minutes.

Sweeten with a little molasses.

Flatulence
Can be due to a fault in the digestive system leading to fermentation of food and the formation of gases. There may be a deficiency of the B vitamins and an inadequate supply of

stomach acids. Food may be eaten too hurriedly, air taken in during a meal, or too much liquid taken with food. An excellent remedy is 'seed tea. Mix equal quantities of fennel seeds, anise seeds and caraway seeds. Take one teaspoonful of the mixture, crush, and put into a cupful of boiling water. Cover, leave to infuse for ten minutes, strain, and drink this warm infusion after a meal.

An infusion of catmint taken cool will help to overcome flatulence: the dose is two tablespoonfuls before each meal. It can be given to infants in teaspoonful doses before or with each feed. Peppermint tea is good too, and so is ginger. If tincture of ginger is available, take up to five drops in a tablespoonful of warm water, especially if feeling chilled. Many of the culinary herbs contain volatile oils which aid digestion, and using these as fresh herbs sprinkled on salads or, dried, used in cooking will reduce or prevent flatulence.

It will be better not to drink with meals, have fruit juices, weak tea or other drinks between meals, chew food well, and eat when relaxed, not when tense or keyed up.

Vitamin B complex will help production of digestive juices and will feed the nervous system. If none of these measures are effective consult a herbal practitioner in order to ascertain the cause of the complaint.

Fractures

A broken bone may be a closed fracture when the skin is intact, or an open fracture when the bone has penetrated the skin. In accidents, when broken bones are suspected, the victim should be taken to hospital as quickly as possible but should not be moved until the injured limb has been stabilized, using the body or other limb as a support.

Comfrey, because of its constituent allantoin, has the property of healing bone tissue. It should be taken as a tea, and when possible its leaves used as a poultice around the injury. Either leaves or root may be prepared as a tea: the leaves covered with boiling water and left, covered, to stand until cold. The liquid is taken in wineglassful doses three or four times daily, and the leaves may be applied as a poultice encased in muslin or fine bandage. This bandage should be kept moist with the liquid, and be changed every twenty-four hours. If the root is used, 1 oz (25g) finely chopped or sliced root is allowed to stand for four hours in 1 pint (0.5 litre) of cold water, strained as required in wineglassful doses three times daily.

At the time of the fracture it might be wise to treat the victim for shock. Give a teaspoonful or so of antispasmodic tincture in warm water, or a drop of Bach Rescue Remedy, every few minutes.

Freckles

Not a health problem, but may be an annoyance. Avoid strong sunshine and apply either lemon juice or a lotion of elder leaves. Cover a few washed elder leaves with boiling water, leave to stand until cool, covered to prevent steam from escaping. Dab this on the freckled area every day.

Gallstones

An excess of cholesterol and bile salts in the gall-bladder leads to the formation of gall-stones. The cause is only too often an over-indulgence in rich foods, lack of exercise and obesity, a vicious circle which needs a change of life-style.

A short fast, followed by a diet from which animal fats have been excluded, in which plenty of lemon and grapefruit juices are taken to stimulate the liver, and preferably a vegetarian diet.

A number of herbal remedies are used by the practitioner to gradually dissolve the stone and to improve function of the liver and gall-bladder in order to prevent any recurrence.

Amongst these is dandelion, which gently stimulates the liver and reduces cholesterol. The fresh young leaves should be mixed with salad greens in the daily salad, and an infusion made by adding 1 oz (25g) of leaves and a similar quantity of chopped root to 2 pints (1 litre) of cold water and allowing to steep for two hours. It is then gradually brought to the boil, held at that point for one minute, then removed from heat and allowed to stand for a further twenty minutes. It should be strained and taken in two wineglassful doses fifteen minutes before each meal.

Gentian root is used also, prepared as a decoction, taken in wineglassful doses shortly before each meal. Chamomile has an influence on the liver; the tea taken between meals is beneficial. Black root, celandine, wild yam, and other remedies in the herbalist's dispensary are used in formulae specific to the individual patient.

Gastric Ulcer

The formation of an ulcer on the wall of the stomach or the duodenum is associated with a certain type of temperament, with stress, irregular hurried meals, and faulty diet. The cause must be attended to by altering diet and also the way of life, if necessary. Herbal teas, both on a regular basis and occasionally to relieve discomfort, will be invaluable. An infusion of meadowsweet will reduce acidity, gentian root taken in two-tablespoonful doses, before meals, will have the dual purpose of influencing liver function and aiding assimilation of food. Chamomile tea influences nervous control of the stomach, relaxing and soothing, easing nausea. It should be taken in wineglassful doses three times daily, with more whenever required.

Slippery elm is essential for all types of gastric disorders, and more so when ulceration has taken place. It has a soothing and healing effect on the stomach lining. Use the slippery elm powder, mixing one teaspoonful to asmooth paste with a little honey, gradually adding a cupful of hot water or milk and water. A little nutmeg may be grated on the surface if desired. This drink should be taken at least twice every day. Comfrey tea is also healing. All herbal teas should be taken warm, at body temperature, when taken for gastric disorders. Golden seal is a most valuable herb for ulcers and other gastric disturbances.

It is often necessary to take nerve remedies to promote a more relaxed state of mind and body before a gastric ulcer can be overcome. Chamomile has already been mentioned. Balm can be very relaxing; it was stated by an ancient herbalist to 'make the heart merry', and has been found particularly helpful for nervous indigestion and nervous colic. Marjoram has an equally good reputation; the fresh herb chopped and sprinkled on salads, the dried herb used in cooking or a cupful taken before or after meals (1/2 teaspoonful to a small teacup of boiling water, covered and left to cool) will reinforce the other remedies.

See Nervous Disorders, for more information.

Gastritis
Inflammation of the stomach is usually due to faulty diet, to bolting large meals often accompanied by alcohol, or to the

effects on the stomach of anxiety, worry, fear or resentment. If not attended to it can eventually lead to a gastric ulcer. A wineglassful of chamomile tea before each meal will soothe the nerves; this may be alternated with the same quantity of avens to stimulate and aid digestion. An infusion of marshmallow leaves taken several times daily in wineglassful doses will soothe an irritated and inflamed stomach lining. Prepare this by adding 1 oz (25g) of the leaves to 1 pint (0.5 litres) of boiling water, and allowing to stand, covered, for ten minutes, then straining the liquid.

Slippery elm should be taken in addition to the herbal teas for its demulcent, soothing properties, both as a drink and in tablet form: Two tablets after meals will ease discomfort.

Slippery elm tablets are made by Potters, Gerard and others.

Diet for both gastritis and gastric ulcer should exclude fried foods, vinegar, pickles, hot spicy foods, large meals, and drinking with meals. Simple small meals on a lacto vegetarian whole food principle should be taken at fairly frequent intervals, chewed well, and only eaten when in a relaxed frame of mind.

Gastro-enteritis

A preparation of equal quantities of oak bark, bayberry bark, agrimony, raspberry leaves and calamus root, taken in teacupful doses every two or three hours will control the inflammation and loose bowel action. Add 1 oz (25g) of the mixed herbs to 1 1/2 pints (0.75 litres) of cold water, heat to boiling point, simmer gently for fifteen minutes and strain when cool. Continue taking a wineglassful three times daily for a further day or two to clear the condition, but not if constipated. Both slippery elm and marshmallow will soothe the irritated tissues, and should be taken two or three times daily in teacupful doses.

No food should be taken during the acute stage, but homemade vegetable soup can be taken two or three times in the day when the symptoms have subsided and the appetite returns, and other foods gradually introduced.

Glandular Fever

A contagious fever mostly confined to children and young people, with temperatures up to 39°C (103°F), and swelling of lymphatic glands in the neck and elsewhere. It will last for about ten days, and a slow convalescence can be expected, with the possibility of subsequent recurrence.

Herbal treatment can alter that!

Rest in bed is imperative until the temperature has returned to normal, although it is advisable to isolate the patient for a week. Frequent herbal teas of yarrow, elderflower, peppermint and clivers in equal quantities should be taken hot to promote perspiration. Add 2oz (50g) of the mixture to 2 pints (1 litre) of boiling water, allow to infuse, covered, for fifteen minutes, and take in wineglassful doses every hour or two until perspiration has taken place and the temperature begins to drop. It can be alternated with sage tea made with one teaspoonful of the crushed leaves and 1/2 pint (0.25 litres) of boiling water, covered closely and infused for fifteen minutes. An excellent tonic during convalescence is a wineglassful of vervain tea taken cold three or four times daily. It has the advantage of slight antibiotic properties. No food should be taken during the fever. Plenty of diluted fruit juices and pure water (i.e., bottled spring water) should be taken as often as desired.

The bowels should be kept open, as in all fevers.

When the appetite returns, take fresh ripe fruits, a little salad and home-made vegetable soups for a few days, gradually introducing wholesome foods to follow a good diet. It is important to build up the general health after an attack of glandular fever to prevent recurrence.

Diagnosis is essential in this condition, as symptoms in the early stages can resemble those of acute leukaemia.

Gout

The intense pain and inflammation in the great toe joint is an indication of a system high in uric acid, usually resulting from excessive intake of meat, rich foods, and - in most cases - alcohol. There will have been a lack of alkaline foods. A family tendency to arthritis may be in the background.

Immediate introduction of salads, plenty of celery and parsley, green leafy vegetables, plus a change over to a near-vegetarian diet will instigate improvement.

An effective remedy is a combination of broom tops, burdock root, dandelion root and meadowsweet, in equal quantities: 1 oz (25g) of the mixture is added to 1 1/2 pints (0.75 litre) of cold water, allowed to stand covered for two hours, then brought to the boil and simmered very gently for two minutes. It should be taken off the heat and left to stand for twenty minutes before straining. The dose is a wineglassful about fifteen minutes before each meal.

Another useful remedy is equal quantities of couch grass, wood betony, sarsaparilla bark and half the quantity of prickly ash bark. Preparation and dosage is as above.

The pain can be relieved by poulticing with comfrey leaves, chamomile flowers or St John's wort. Cover the chosen herb with boiling water, leave to stand for twenty minutes, then apply the herb encased in gauze or fine muslin. Keep moist with the liquid, change every few hours.

Follow a light diet during an attack of gout, avoiding meat, vinegar, pickles, sugar and fried foods. Eat plenty of watercress, and have raw cherries when in season, up to 1/2lb (250g) daily.

Gravel

Kidney stones are formed of either uric acid crystals, calcium oxalate, calcium phosphate or a mixture. They may be related to a lack of fresh vegetables and vitamin A or to some metabolic disorder frequently associated with the parathyroid gland. The herbal practitioner will direct treatment to correcting dietary imbalance, and will use herbs to improve metabolism and to dissolve the stones, eliminating the broken-down substances. Gravel root and clivers both clear uric acid from the system, and parsley piert, known to an earlier generation of herbalists as parsley breakstone, willgradually clear the stones from the urinary system. A wineglassful of these herbs, either alone or combined together will be very helpful, but the condition should be treated professionally.

Gum and Mouth Problems

A healthy diet leads to a healthy mouth, chewing raw salads, apples and other crisp fruits cleans the teeth and has an almost antiseptic effect in the mouth, inhibiting bacteria and the depositing of tartar on the teeth.

The most useful remedy for sore, inflamed gums is tincture of myrrh, which should be massaged thoroughly with the fingertip into the gums each day. It has an astringent and anti-bacterial action, and regular use will strengthen the gums. It can also be used on mouth ulcers.

Other astringent remedies can be prepared as normal infusions and used daily as a mouthwash. These include agrimony, bistort, potentilla (which is good for pyorrhoea) and the more soothing marshmallow. If gumboils occur, swab them several times daily with blackberry leaf tea, and drink a wineglassful two or three times daily. An infusion of centaury herb used as a mouthwash will also relieve inflamed gums. Slippery elm has helped ease gingivitis, the powder mixed to a paste with water, applied, and held in the mouth for a few minutes.

Weleda have produced a comprehensive range of preparations from herbs, essential oils and other natural substances in the form of toothpaste, gargle and mouthwash.

Easy to use and pleasant in taste, they will help to keep the mouth and gums healthy.

Haemorrhage

Internal bleeding, whether from the lungs, stomach or bowels, must be dealt with professionally. A number of herbs have astringent properties and can be used to staunch some bleeding quite quickly. For example the superficial bleeding of cuts or surface wounds will respond quickly to the application of fresh yarrow leaves, avens leaves or woundwort. Nettles have good astringent properties too: used as an infusion they can be applied on compresses.

Cranesbill root is an effective astringent: the powdered root can be sprinkled on a wound or infused to be used as a compress.

Recurrent bursting of blood vessels under the skin, petechiae, is a sign of weakened capillaries and deficiency of vitamin C. Rutin tablets and at least 500mg of the vitamin daily will strengthen the tiny blood vessels.

See also Nosebleed.

Haemorrhoids

These small painful swellings in the anus are formed by restriction in the upward flow of blood from the rectum, causing veins to become permanently distended, resulting from pressure in the abdomen - pregnancy, liver congestion and constipation being the most common causes. The haemorrhoids will be either internal, causing heat and itching in the rectum, or external, causing an aching feeling of pressure and fullness. The first remedy to consider is lesser celandine (pilewort) which should be applied two or three times daily, certainly after a bowel movement. It will relieve and reduce the haemorrhoids.

Distilled witch-hazel is gently astringent, cooling and soothing and will also shrink them. Several herbs are useful both to apply and to take internally as an infusion, such as blackberry leaves, cranesbill, rtormentil and dock. In addition, Heath & Heather have a combined treatment, pilewort ointment and tablets, as has Roberts of Bristol.

Both Napier's and Gerard have either ointment or tablets.

The use of any of these remedies, associated with a changed diet which will ensure freedom from constipation, and any necessary treatment for other local conditions which could contribute, will overcome haemorrhoids permanently.

Hair

The condition of the hair is a good indication of health; if shining and luxuriant it needs no extra care. Lifeless, thinning hair points to the need for a diet rich in silica, B vitamins, fresh fruits and vegetables, vitamins A and C, so diet and general health must be improved.

Sage tea is a good hair and scalp tonic for brunettes; a little rubbed well into the scalp each day, and a warm infusion used as a final rinse when shampooing will gradually improve the quality and texture of the hair. Chamomile infusion may be used in the same way for blondes.

Rosemary is a good general hair tonic; an infusion can be taken in wineglassful doses as a general nerve tonic and can also be used to rub well into the scalp daily and when washing the hair. An infusion of comfrey leaves, elderflowers or burdock root will improve dry hair, whilst an oily scalp needs lavender herb. In both instances, the liquid should be rubbed into the scalp daily. An infusion of nettles brushed or combed into the hair each day will add shine.

Almond oil massaged all over the scalp before shampooing will improve the scalp. Many of these herbs are available in preparations for the hair, as shampoos, rinses, etc., and can be obtained from health food stores.

Halitosis

Seek the cause of bad breath, which may be due to dental problems, digestive disorders, constipation, or certain foods, and deal with the problem directly. In the meantime, chew Heath & Heather's chlorophyll tablets, a sprig or two of parsley, a few mint leaves, a sprig of basil, rosemary or thyme. Make an infusion of lemon verbena herb or of lavender and use it as a mouthwash. Rub one or two sage leaves round the teeth and gums. Use Weleda toothpaste and mouthwash.

Hay Fever

An early sensitivity to milk protein, coupled with a diet low in fresh raw fruits and salads can be one of the causes of hay fever. Perseverance in taking herbal teas, reinforced by the measures under the heading Catarrh (page 40) will, in the majority of cases, overcome the condition.

A good combination of remedies for hay fever is 102 (25g) each of yarrow herb, wood betony and eyebright, added to 2 pints (1 litre) of boiling water, covered and allowed to infuse for ten minutes. The dose is a wineglassful night and morning for a moderate attack, increasing to every few hours when at its worst. Another useful herbal tea is equal quantities of eyebright, lungwort and golden rod. Mix well together, add a heaped teaspoonful to a teacupful of boiling water, cover and infuse for ten minutes. Strain, and drink whilst still warm. This may be taken three times daily. Children suffering from hay fever would have a appropriately smaller dose (see Childrens' Ailments, for details).

The action of these herbs will be reinforced by taking a vitamin C tablet and biochemic tissue salts (either ferr. phos. or the hay fever combination) alternately between the herbal remedies at regular intervals. Start treatment well before the hay fever season, and build up resistance during the year by having a diet low in dairy products, but abundant in raw vegetables and salads, and by taking at least 500mg vitamin C daily. If hay fever does not respond to this approach it would be wise to consult a herbal practitioner.

Heart Disorders

The heart muscle continuously pumps approximately six litres of blood throughout the miles of blood vessels in the body, and is capable of working constantly throughout a long life, but is dependent for its integrity and good health upon efficient working of the liver and kidneys and upon healthy blood. It can be affected by digestive problems, by hormones, e.g., thyroid gland disorders, and by 'nerves'

It is vulnerable to the suppressive drugs used in the treatment of many diseases and to the stimulants of coffee, alcohol, tobacco and strong tea. Apart from congenital heart disease, damaged valves or other structural faults, treatment of heart problems begins in childhood with good nutrition and natural treatment of any childhood ailments.

The right food has to be the foundation of any treatment of heart condition. Animal fats and dairy products which can cause liver and gall-bladder problems and lead to 'furring up' of blood vessels, thus making it harder for the blood to be pumped round the body, should be replaced by vegetable oils, soya milk and plant milk. Excessive carbohydrates (refined sugar and starches) which cast an extra burden on the liver and provide no nutrition other than calorific energy, should be reduced in quantity and replaced by honey, whole-wheat and whole grains, and very little cane sugar. A high-protein, high-salt diet creates problems for the kidneys. A semi-vegetarian diet will ease that burden, meat being replaced by nuts, pulses and seeds, a little cheese and up to three eggs per week.

There are many herbs used by the herbal practitioner to treat heart conditions: hawthorn for its gentle control of tachycardia, its ability to strengthen heart muscle and to gently reduce raised blood pressure: lily of the valley for its action in correcting arrythmia, of strengthening the heart action, motherwort for its sedative effect on fast beating heart associated with 'nerves', a gentle tonic for women in particular. Many other remedies are used according to the individual patient's needs.

Heart problems should not be dealt with until professional

diagnosis and treatment has been sought, nor should drug treatment be stopped without the guidance of the doctor or other physician.

Heartburn

An excess of acid-forming foods, or over-production of hydrochloric acid in the stomach gives rise to the burning discomfort rising from the stomach after a meal, occasionally with eructation of liquid into the throat.

Meadowsweet herb is alkaline and a wineglassful sipped after a meal will counteract the acidity. Slippery elm tablets taken after food will also give relief, as will Potter's acidosis tablets. The cause of heartburn should be found and treated.

Hepatitis

Inflammation of the liver arises as a result of a virus or other infection. Rest in bed is essential during the early stages. Pure water with a trace of lemon or grapefruit juice (unsweetened) may be taken as thirst dictates. Chamomile tea will gradually allay the nausea. No food must be taken until the appetite is keen. Herbal teas of such remedies as black root, fringe tree bark and gentian root, combined with some wild indigo for its anti-virus properties, will help.

The bowels should be kept open either by enemas or by gentle laxatives (see Constipation).

Convalescence can take a month or two, and it will be wise to avoid fats, fried foods, sugar and alcohol for some time after that. Verbena tea during convalescence will aid digestion and the liver, and will act as a gentle tonic. The condition should be under the care of a practitioner.

Hernia

Excessive or careless lifting of heavy objects can lead to the protrusion of a loop of the intestines through a weakened layer of muscle in the abdomen. This should receive the attention of a practitioner, but as an interim measure a poultice of comfrey leaves will give some relief. Even more helpful, a compress made from oak bark applied daily will strengthen the weak tissues. Simmer 2 oz (50g) of the finely chopped bark for ten minutes in 1pint (0.5 litre) of water, strain when cool, and use to soak a pad of lint or cotton fabric. This should be bound firmly in place and changed every twenty-four hours.

Hiccups

This often embarrassing complaint is caused by spasmodic contraction of the diaphragm (the dome-shaped sheet of muscle which divides the abdomen from the chest). It will usually respond to chewing a few mint leaves, a few dill seeds, or to frequent sips of catmint tea taken hot (one teaspoonful to a teacupful of boiling water, covered and allowed to infuse for five minutes). If none of these are successful place a teaspoonful of crushed dill seeds in a large teacup, add a little boiling water, stir and infuse for a few minutes. Strain, and make the quantity up toa teacupful with cold water. Take a deep breath; bend forward to sip the liquid as quickly as you can from the opposite side of the cup. Take twenty sips whilst holding the breath and the hiccups should be cured.

Hoarseness

An infusion of marshmallow leaves and flowers with honey added to taste taken in wineglassful doses three or four times daily will soothe the throat. Frequent gargling will help to reduce inflammation and return the voice to normal. A good gargle is prepared by adding 1oz (25g) of agronomy herb to 1 1/2 pints (0.75 litre) of boiling water and simmering gently until reduced to 1pint (0.5 litre). Strain when cold and gargle with a small quantity as many as ten times in the day for quick results. An infusion of fennel (either seeds or leaves) can be used in the same way. The seeds should be crushed before being infused.

Hyperactivity

Incessantly on the go, quick-thinking, irritable, with temper tantrums, poor sleep, poor concentration and a finicky appetite, hyperactivity in children is becoming more common.

The herbal practitioner has a number of remedies which are sedative to the nervous system, non-addictive and perfectly safe for children, and these are successful in the majority of cases. Diet must be reviewed, a great deal of research has been carried out in America which shows that these children are sensitive to food additives - colourings, preservatives and flavourings - and that when put on a diet totally free from additives and very low in sugar they improve rapidly. Apractitioner should be consulted, and help with diet sought.

Hypoglycaemia

Undue fatigue, tremulousness, depression, headaches, irritability and other 'nerve' symptoms can be due to low blood sugar. All carbohydrates are converted during the processes of digestion to a simple sugar, glucose, of which about two teaspoonful is in the bloodstream and the rest is stored in muscles and elsewhere for immediate use. All the body needs glucose, especially the muscles and brain.

When sugar is eaten the pancreas produces insulin to control the amount in the bloodstream. In a diet which contains large amounts of starch and sugar the pancreas can eventually become over-stimulated. Too much insulin is secreted, creating too lowa level of blood sugar.

The herbal practitioner has remedies for this problem and will use them in conjunction with changes in diet. One useful herb is liquorice root, for its influence on the adrenal glands, involved in the process, and the pancreas. Either the sticks of the root peeled and prepared as a decoction or the solid juices can be used. Peel 2 oz (50g) of the sticks, add to 2 pints (1 litre) of boiling water and simmer for fifteen minutes. Leave to cool. If using the solid juice take a piece about 3 inches (7cm) in length, break it up and dissolve in ½ pint (0.25 litres) of hot water. The dose of either is a wineglassful three times daily, remembering that liquorice is a gentle laxative.

Remedies for the liver and digestion to normalize the appetite and reduce the craving for sweet foods that is often part of the condition would be a supportive treatment, and would include gentian root, agrimony and black root.

Diet should exclude completely all refined carbohydrates and should consist of mixed proteins, whole grains, nuts, sunflower seeds, millet, cheeses, yogurt and plenty of salads and vegetables. The only sugar to be taken should be the natural sugars in fruits. The herbal practitioner will of course advise on this condition, and should be consulted.

Impetigo

This contagious skin condition requires strict hygiene to prevent transmission to other family members. Echinacea tablets should be given daily, and a lotion prepared from marigold flowers, fresh when possible, should be applied frequently. The petals from a dozen marigold heads should be simmered gently for five minutes and left to infuse for a further ten; ½ pint (0.25 litre) of water will make a lotion of moderate strength. When cool, add ten drops of tincture of iodine. Calendula cream or ointment can be used, but the fresh infusion will be more quickly effective.

Impotence

The cause may be a lowered level of health and vitality, perhaps following an illness or a long period of stress, or may be due to deficient diet, or of emotional origin. The cause should be ascertained and dealt with.

Various remedies are available to improve general vitality, amongst them are ginseng, which influences all systems of the body, Roberts' Super-tonic or Strength tablets, Napier's Strength tablets. Both Heath & Heather's Tonic and Nerve mixture and Potter's Neuralax relieve the effects of stress.

Vitamin E should be taken, either alone or combined with ginseng. A wholesome nutritious diet, which includes whole grains (the sources of vitamin E) and plenty of fresh raw foods, outdoor exercise and lots of fresh air, will all contribute to improvement.

Incontinence

May be caused by interference in the nerve supply to bladder muscles by disease or injury; in old age it is due to weakened muscles. There are cases in which the damage is too advanced to be helped. One remedy which has proved to be very helpful and is worth trying is horsetail; 1oz (25g) taken in one tablespoonful doses three times daily. Raspberry leaf tea, for its astringency and its properties of strengthening pelvic muscles has also been used for this problem. A small teacupful of the normal infusion taken night and morning should be adequate, but can be increased.

Infectious Disorders

The wide range of infections to which the human being is subject can hardly be discussed in a few sentences. Some of the comments under Fevers will be applicable.

Garlic is a superb and powerful herbal antibiotic. Taken regularly, especially during winter, it will gradually build up resistance against infection. Eucalyptus is another antibiotic remedy. The tree was known as the 'fever tree' because of its effectiveness against infections and fevers.

Boil 1oz (25g) of the leaves for one minute in 2 pints (1 Litre) of water, leave to stand (still covered) for ten minutes and then strain. The dose is a small teacupful three or four times daily to combat virus and other infections. The warm infusion can be inhaled for influenza which is affecting the lungs. Bayberry bark is used by herbal practitioners for various infections and is incorporated in a number of remedies. Tincture of wild indigo, taken in small doses every two or three hours will gradually overcome the most persistent virus. Up to five drops in about a dessertspoonful of cold water is an adequate dose.

Infertility

Examinations and tests are necessary to discover the cause of infertility. Attend to general health, include wheat germ and plenty of raw foods in the daily diet, take vitamin B complex and at least 200m of vitamin E daily. Learn relaxation, as tension itself has been known to inhibit conception, and have a relaxed attitude during love-making, not a tense 'will it happen this time' approach.

Balm tea is of benefit to tense women, and influences pelvic and uterine muscles, relaxing the tensions which cause cramp-like pains at period time. A wineglassful of the normal infusion, which has been allowed to infuse for ten minutes, can be taken three to six times daily. Feverfew leaves provide a good tonic for the uterus. Some of the properties are lost when subject to heat, so six fresh leaves should be taken daily with salad or part of a salad sandwich, together with two tablespoonfuls each night and morning of an infusion made by adding ½ oz (12.5g) of the leaves to 1 pint (0.5 litre) of cold water. It should be left to stand for an hour, in sunshine if possible, warmed gently to blood heat, and then taken off the heat and left to cool. Ginseng capsules will also be beneficial.

Inflammation

Inflammation is the body's local protection response to some form of injury or destructive element. It should be helped, not suppressed.

Cold compresses should be applied; a soft cotton cloth wrung out in plain cold water (not ice-cold) or a cold infusion of marshmallow leaves or plantain leaves should be applied over the area and replaced as soon as it is warm.

The cause of the inflammation should be found and dealt with. Echinacea tablets, infusion of burdock or small doses of wild indigo root, may each be indicated according to the cause of the inflammation.

Influenza

Do not regard influenza as merely a very bad cold; the virus can be powerful, can lie dormant in body cells where antibiotics cannot attack it, and will emerge to give rise to another, usually milder, attack.

As much rest as possible should be taken, at least two days in bed or until temperature is normal. Herbal teas should be taken everyone or two hours, diluted fruit juices or hot lemon and honey being taken frequently to allay thirst. At the first sign of influenza, composition essence or some herbal influenza mixture should be taken in hot water, every two hours, and boneset tea, a wineglassful as hot as can be taken, for the aching limbs, catmint tea, also hot, for restlessness, pleurisy root if the chest and lungs are involved, sage tea if the throat is sore.

To make an infusion of sage add 1/2oz (12.5g) of sage to just under 2 pints (1 litre) of boiling water, simmer for five minutes and leave to stand for five or ten minutes before straining. This infusion may be used as a gargle, and some honey added to the remainder to be taken in wineglassful doses as required. Sage has some antiseptic properties. A good combination of herbs for influenza is equal quantities 1 of elderflowers, yarrow, boneset, white horehound and peppermint herb, mixed well together. Add two tablespoonfuls to 1 pint (0.5 litre) of boiling water, allow to stand for ten minutes. Take half this mixture hot at bedtime, and take the remainder cool during the following day.

Vervain tea is excellent to take as a tonic after influenza, more so when depression is an aftermath.

The herbal practitioner has various other remedies which can be used to treat influenza. A number of remedies are easily available, such as elderflower, peppermint and composition essence, and others.

If influenza is a recurrent problem it would be wise to attend to general health, to take adequate vitamin supplement to build up resistance to infection and have adequate rest, exercise and fresh air.

Insect Bites and Stings

To try to keep insects away rub the exposed skin with the moisture from crushed elder leaves, or tansy leaves, with lavender oil, or with a strong infusion of either lavender, rosemary, sage, wormwood or St John's Wort. A bunch of basil herb will keep flies away. Herbs can be hung in small bunches in wardrobes, or placed in small muslin bags in cupboards and drawers to discourage moths. Herbs suitable for this are sage, southernwood, rosemary, balm, and summer savoury.

To apply to insect bites and stings: plantain leaves, crushed to express the juice, or infused in boiling water; hyssop leaves, crushed; rosemary, either fresh leaves or an infusion; oil or essence of lavender or of pennyroyal.

Bee stings should be dealt with by pulling ou t the sting and then dabbing the spot with distilled witch-hazel, tincture of marigold or calendula (marigold) cream.

Wasp stings should have cider vinegar or ordinary vinegar applied. If there is the need to take some herbal tea after a bite or sting, an infusion of balm, borage, broom, echinacea, fennel seeds or gentian root would help ease the discomfort: balm for the nerves, and the other herbs to clear poisons from the bloodstream.

Insomnia

'Sleep that knits up the ravelled sleeve of care' is sometimes too elusive. A warm bath at bedtime to which a strong infusion of hops has been added will create a pleasant relaxed drowsiness and usually leads on to sleep. The type of restless wakefulness with much dreaming will respond to wood betony. A teaspoonful added to a teacupful of boiling water, infused in a small teapot for five minutes with honey added to taste, should be sipped slowly when in a warm bed. Insomnia may be due to worries and anxieties and for such causes herbal teas should be taken during the day, in addition to the bedtime dose. Skullcap, valerian and passiflora in equal quantities are a good mixture for this purpose, infused for ten minutes and taken in wineglassful doses after meals and at bedtime. Allow 1oz (25g) to 1pint (0.5 litre) of boiling water. An alternative is ½ oz (12.5g) each of hops, valerian and passiflora. Add to 1pint (0.5 litre) boiling water, cover and leave to cool. Dosage is as above.

There are many prepared remedies for sleeplessness: Napier's Passiflor tablets, Weleda Avena Sativa compound, Heath & Heather's Quiet Night tablets, Potter's Ana-sed, Roberts' Calmanite, and Gerard Valerian compound tablets. There is a good range of herbal non-addictive tablets from which to choose. Some of them, Lane's Kalms, for example, can be taken during the day without making one sleepy as well as at bedtime, and have the effect of relieving the strains and stresses of everyday living. Calcium may be helpful too, stress and some drugs deplete the nerves of vital calcium. A calcium lactate tablet (300mg) taken two or three times daily will remedy this. _

A warm bath at bedtime will often induce sleep. One containing an infusion of hops will create a delightful drowsy sensation. Up to 1 oz (25g) can be infused for ten minutes before adding to the bath, or the hops may be added in a muslin bag. The same effect is achieved with lavender or rosemary. Agood handful of either, simmered gently for about ten minutes then strained and added to the bath water will be adequate. A wineglassful of the normal infusion (1 teaspoonful to a teacupful) may be sipped warm when in a warm bed. Wild lettuce has a soporific effect, the cultivated varieties a little less so, but a sandwich oflettuce and onion at bedtime could be helpful.

American research has shown that onions contain a constituent which relaxes the nerves and brain and can help overcome insomnia. A snack about half an hour before bedtime - salad sandwich, cheese and whole-wheat biscuits or similar light foods containing the amino acid L-tryptophan will in many cases lead to a good sleep. L-tryptophan is a precursor of a sleep-inducing substance found in the brain, serotonin.

For those who are able, a brisk walk or short spell of reasonably vigorous exercise, sufficient to bring about a natural tiredness, taken shortly before retiring to bed is the answer. For others, a few minutes spent doing deep breathing exercises, relaxing the body thoroughly, and indulging in some day-dreaming about pleasant memories will be effective. If wakeful during the night, getting up to make a cup of herbal tea and reading or sewing for a short time instead oflying in bed trying not to toss and turn, can be more relaxing. Chamomile, lime blossom or weak lavender tea will be appropriate at such a time. When there has been daytime stress or mental over-activity the adrenal glands are often stimulated into activity in the early hours, and the effect of their production of adrenalin can last for two hours. At the end of that time there is the feeling of something being switched off and drowsiness creeps over one just before drifting into sleep.

Irritable Bowel Syndrome

The following herbs have been found effective in controlling the condition: 1 oz (25g) each of meadowsweet, marshmallow root, plantain leaves and bayberry powder, 1.2 oz (12.5g) each of hops, chamomile flowers and prickly ash bark. Mix well, add 2 oz (50g) to 2 pints (1 litre) of boiling water, simmer gently for fifteen minutes, take off the heat and leave to cool. Strain, and take a wineglassful before meals. An additional tisane of chamomile flowers can be taken two or three times dailybetween meals. Slippery elm will be soothing - at least three cupsful daily will benefit.

Do not have stimulants such as strong tea, coffee, alcohol, vinegar, pickles, curries, and follow a semi-vegetarian diet, avoiding pork, ham and bacon.

Jaundice

The yellow pigmentation of skin and eyes occurs as the result of excessive bile pigment in the blood-stream, caused by infection, blockage of the bile-ducts or damage to the liver cells. Treatment should be given by a practitioner as diagnosis of the cause is essential.

In the meantime herbal teas of agrimony, fumitory, gentian root, yellow dock root or dandelion root would be of some help. The normal infusion of the herbs, or decoction of roots, taken in wineglassful doses three or four times daily can be used if no treatment is available.

No food should be taken, only fresh grapes at mealtimes and plenty of lemon or grapefruit juice well diluted with pure (bottled) water, until normal colour returns.

Kidney Disorders

Kidney disease must be attended to by a practitioner, but some disorders can respond quickly to appropriate herbal teas. If there is any known kidney disease present, or if there are recurrent symptoms of kidney problems it is essential to avoid fluoridated water completely and to have a low-protein or vegetarian diet.

Dandelion root is a gentle diuretic and stimulant to the kidneys. Horsetail is useful in any inflammatory condition, it helps to dissolve renal stones and is used by the herbal practitioner in cases of bed-wetting. Uva ursi is a good remedy for most kidney and bladder problems, especially when there is backache or a tendency to rheumatism.

Meadowsweet should be included in the teas in such conditions. Both gravel root and clivers will also help dissolve renal stones and help promote the flow of urine.

Agrimony, when combined with the other remedies will tone the mucous membrane lining of the urinary system.

There are of course a number of proprietary remedies.

The diet could include young dandelion leaves in salad, parsley, asparagus and grapes. Avoid coffee, even decaffeinated, as it is an irritant to kidney tissue.

See also Bladder and Urinary Problems, and Cystitis.

Laryngitis

A localized virus infection or the spread of infection from the nose and throat, this dry sore throat with an irritating cough and hoarseness can be quite unpleasant.

Make an infusion of sage, thyme and marjoram, one teaspoonful each to ½ pint (0.25 litre) of boiling water, add one peeled liquorice stick, and simmer very gently for only two minutes. Take off the heat, allow to cool and strain. Take one tablespoonful three times daily, and an extra spoonful occasionally to ease the cough. Either sage or thyme may be used alone; one teaspoonful to a teacupful of boiling water, used as a gargle. No honey or liquorice should be added to this. A cold compress outside the throat can help reduce the inflammation and soreness. (See Tonsillitis, for directions.) Take care with diet, avoiding dairy products. Eat plenty of onions for their antiseptic properties. One day on nothing other than boiled onions at mealtimes would do a great deal of good. Drinks should be garlic honey in hot water or lemon juice and honey in hot water. The garlic honey is prepared by slicing two large cloves of garlic finely and stirring them into 4 oz (100g) of liquid honey. Cover the dish closely and leave to stand overnight. Take a teaspoonful of the honey to each cupful of hot water.

Another useful remedy is lavender. Infuse 1 oz (25g) of the flowers and flowering tips in 2 pints (1 litre) of boiling water in a covered vessel for five minutes. Take a wineglassful three times daily, and inhale the warm infusion several times. Lavender is antiseptic and tonic – thus useful in all infections of the respiratory tract.

Lassitude (See Debility)

Lethargy
A normal state of recuperation after a serious illness or a prolonged spell of overwork and stress. For good remedies see

Convalescence and Debility. If it is prolonged, professional advice must be sought.

Liver

A healthy liver is a primary need in maintaining good health or overcoming disease. Its many complex functions can be upset by drugs, excessive alcohol, tobacco, carbohydrates, food additives, and by infections; a congested or damaged liver can contribute to a lowered standard of health and to diseases of other organs.

Blood filters through the liver at a rate of 3 pints (1.5 litres) every minute, and during that minute the liver neutralizes any toxins present in the blood, retains an appropriate quantity of iron and glucose for storage and converts fats, proteins and carbohydrates into their final stage of digestion for use in the body. Bile, antibodies, enzymes and seven of the ten proteins required for blood clotting are manufactured in the liver from nutrients absorbed from blood. The liver produces over one thousand enzymes, the compounds of which are used throughout the body in innumerable activities. Loss of certain of these leads to disorders of digestion and assimilation. Liver disorders are in the background of biliousness, poor appetite and irregular bowel action.

Dandelion is a fine remedy, a slow, mild tonic which gently stimulates liver function and improves digestion and assimilation. It can be taken in combination with meadowsweet and fringetree bark, in equal quantities, the usual decoction. Take a wineglassful three times daily.

This will quickly control a bilious attack. No food should be taken until a good healthy appetite returns. Dandelion can also be combined with equal quantities of centaury, wild carrot, vervain, marshmallow root and senna leaves.

Add 2 oz (50g) of the mixture to 2 pints (1 litre) of cold water, bring to the boil and simmer very gently for fifteen minutes, leave to cool and then strain. Take three times daily in wineglassful doses. This will gently stimulate liver function, help to eliminate impurities through the kidneys and will aid digestion. If senna leaves cannot be obtained the pods may be used instead, but half the quantity should be used. Agrimony is another useful herb for the liver, but should not be used if there is constipation. It is astringent, a good tonic for chronic liver disorders. The herbal practitioner has many more herbs which he uses in liver conditions.

Diet should be adjusted to eliminate fatty, fried foods, sugar should be kept to the minimum and foods should be fresh and unprocessed.

Lumbago

A name simply meaning pain in the lumbar region of the back, lumbago usually occurs suddenly as the result of some vigorous activity. The pain is caused by strained muscle fibres or an excessive accumulation of acid in the muscles. A warm bath will usually provide relief, especially if a handful of nettles is added to the bath. If the pain has not eased after a night's sleep the back should be rubbed well two or three times during the day with a good liniment

- Potter's Nine rubbing oils, Olbas oil, Weleda massage balm, or any other good herbal compound. Take remedies to help eliminate acids from the body. The herbal teas, given under Bladder or Kidney headings, would be helpful, or Roberts' Buchu backache compound, Heath & Heather's lumbago mixture or others. There is no shortage of effective herbal treatment for lumbago.

Avoid red meat, red wine and acid-forming foods. Have a very light diet, with plenty of salads, celery, green leafy vegetables, and drink lots of orange juice. If the lumbago persists in spite of these measures an osteopath or herbal practitioner would be of great help.

Lung Disorders

There are many herbs which are effective for lung diseases: lungwort, comfrey, garlic, liquorice, wild cherry, mullein, mallow, to mention only a few of the most useful. Self treatment is not recommended and a professional diagnosis must be sought. It is, however, the experience of all herbal practitioners that treatment with herbal medicines in the early stages of bronchial or lung problems, before the disease has become established and before vitality has been undermined by antibiotics and other drugs, can in most cases effect at least a good improvment and at best a total cure.

A good herbal tea, which will be soothing to irritated lung tissue and will help clear phlegm, which can be taken in conjunction with any other treatment, is 1oz (25g) each of cornfrey root (finely sliced), liquorice root (peeled and chopped), wild cherry bark and marshmallow root, simmered gently for fifteen minutes in 2 pints (1 litre) of water. While this is simmering, infuse 1/2 oz (12.5g) each of coltsfoot, hyssop and lungwort in 1/2 pint (0.25 litres) of boiling water, cover and leave to cool. Strain this through very fine cloth or a paper coffee filter to prevent the fine down in the coltsfoot from irritating the throat. Mix the two liquids together and drink a wineglassful three or four times each day. The dose taken at bedtime could be heated for a more effective influence on the lungs.

Tobacco smoking, whether cigarette or pipe, is a bad habit at any time. When bronchial or lung conditions are present it is senseless and could be suicidal. Smoking has contributed to lung cancer, chronic bronchitis, emphysema, tuberculosis and other lung conditions, to coronary heart disease, cancer of the throat, mouth and oesophagus and that (not surprisingly) it tends to shorten life.

Diet is crucial; milk and dairy products are best avoided and replaced by plantmilk or soya milk, and plenty of raw fresh salads and vegetables will help clear catarrh and phlegm and will increase the body's vitality. Vitamin C will help build up resistance against infection and will have a tonic, healing effect on lung tissues. Some is taken in raw foods but sufficient food cannot be eaten to provide a therapeutic dose; at least 500mg should be taken each day, double that amount during severe illness. Vitamin A has a good influence on the mucous lining of the body organs and will also build resistance to infections.

It is the vitamin given during infections such as pneumonia, measles and others.

Fresh air and deep breathing exercises can help lung conditions. An exercise which can be practised daily and increased in duration and capacity is diaphragmatic breathing; resting the hands on the abdomen below the ribs and pushing the hands upward as the breath is taken in, allowing the hands to sink downwards on exhaling.

Take half a dozen deep breaths, breathing out as long as possible, pause for a few minutes of normal breathing, then take a further six breaths. A second daily exercise is practised whilst walking, inhaling for a certain number of strides, holding the breath and then exhaling for the same number, gradually increasing the strides taken whilst breathing in, holding and breathing out.

Lymphatic Glands

There are over 500 of these glands in the body, comprising a system which plays a primary part in defending the body against infection. The glands become enlarged and painful, for example the tonsils, which consist of a number of lymph glands, herald a cold or influenza with a sore throat.

The herbal practitioner has a number of remedies which assist the lymph glands in their function, in addition to anti-viral and antibiotic remedies to combat infection.

Roberts' Echinacea tablets and Gerard Blue Flag Root tablets are prescribed to cleanse the lymphatic system.

During the course of any infectious disease, the patient should fast on pure water and fruit juices, or follow a very limited diet, but prolonged fasting should not be undertaken by the inexperienced without the care of a practitioner who understands fasting. Food taken when suffering from an acute illness hinders the body in its attempts to clear the disease from the system. No attempt should be made to treat chronically enlarged glands; medical advice must be sought and a diagnosis obtained.

Malnutrition

This nutritional disorder may be due to an insufficient or unbalanced diet, or to a fault in the digestive system which inhibits the assimilation of food.

Remedies can be given to improve appetite and digestion - gentian root, dandelion root; and remedies to assist the liver - black root, fringe tree bark, with a trace of ginger or capsicum. The formula must be an individual one, to serve specific needs. The ever-useful chamomile tea could be taken to support the digestive remedies, peppermint tea would be useful and so would antispasmodic tincture. Two herbs could be taken specifically to assist in a more nutritious way, alfalfa, as a tea or - if the herb can be grown - chopped and mixed with salad each day. The second herb useful in this way is Iceland moss. One teaspoonful to a cupful of hot water, with honey, maple syrup or a little molasses added for flavour, should be taken daily, a pinch of nutmeg or cloves being added occasionally.

Mastitis

This painful inflammation of the breast, which fluctuates during the menstrual cycle, until it can in some cases become chronic, almost always responds well to herbal treatment.

It is advisable to consult a practitioner for medication, although gentle application of distilled witch-hazel or bathing with an infusion of marshmallow flowers and leaves will give some relief.

There has been recent evidence that caffeine shows some association with increase in cystic growths in the breast. Caffeine is, of course, present in coffee, tea, chocolate, cola and similar drinks. It would be sensible to avoid these beverages during treatment and for some time afterwards, to help clear the mastitis thoroughly.

Measles

Most infectious fevers respond well to herbal treatment, which is directed to assisting the body to use its natural defence forces. Rest in bed, with plenty of diluted fruit drinks and herbal teas, will clear measles quickly without risk of ear or chest infection as a sequel.

Equal quantities of clivers, meadowsweet and elderflowers, mixed well, should be added to boiling water, 1 oz (25g) to 1 pint (0.5 litre) allowed to infuse for ten minutes, then strained. The dose is a wineglassful every three hours for a child of ten, half dose for a child of six or younger.

Drink plenty of liquids, but no milk, and do not eat any food except fresh ripe fruits for the two or three days of the rash. The spots may be bathed with the normal infusion of elderflowers.

Memory

Apoor memory is usually due to failure in concentration on the matter in hand, to anxiety, poor circulation to the brain, or to a lowered level of general health coupled with poor diet. A teacupful of sage tea, taken regularly at night and in the morning, will improve the memory, appetite and general well-being if persisted with. A teaspoonful of the crushed dried leaves or five or six fresh leaves to ½ pint (0.25 litre) boiling water, covered closely and left to stand overnight, will provide the day's dose. Rosemary, 'for remembrance', has also been found very helpful when taken regularly, it is a general stimulant to nerves, liver and digestive system. A wineglassful taken before meals will serve its purpose. Add 1oz (25g) of the herb to 1 pint (0.5 litre) of boiling water, cover and infuse for ten minutes.

If taken hot it will promote perspiration in chills and influenza. Balm, taken in wineglassful doses two or three times daily will be beneficial to the nervous system and memory. Infuse as for rosemary. The herb holy thistle has a powerful influence on the blood vessels and will improve circulation to the brain. Add 1oz (25g) of the finely chopped herb to 1pint (0.5 litre) of cold water, heat to boiling point and simmer very gently for two minutes. Sweeten with a little honey. Take a small wineglassful night and morning to improve circulation, memory and to relieve depression.

Do not take holy thistle during pregnancy.

It is necessary to build up health by good nutrition, including vitamin B complex. Make sure the B complex includes choline. This substance is a precursor of acetylcholine, manufactured in the body to ensure efficient functioning of nerve impulses in the brain. Tests have shown improved memory after daily doses of choline as little as 10mg. Choline is present in vegetables, meat and lecithin and is manufactured in the body if other B vitamins and lecithin are taken. A good diet should become a way of living - adequate rest, regular exercise in the fresh air and deep breathing to get plenty of oxygen into the blood-stream, are all part of the memory game!

Meniere's Disease

This persistent and often distressing condition can in some instances respond to a combination of chlorophyll tablets, garlic and liver remedies. The disease is cited in the inner ear, producing attacks of intense vertigo and vomiting, which may last several hours. Each case needs individual treatment and should be under the care of a practitioner.

Diet must include plenty of fresh green vegetables and must exclude sugar and salt. It may be advisable to avoid milk. Vitamin B has helped some sufferers, the B complex plus additional B6.

Menopause

The menopause is a natural function and should be accepted as such, not feared. Abnormal or excessive symptoms often arise because of a stressful life, causing increased hormonal imbalance, years of faulty nutrition, overweight and bad posture leading to undue pressure on pelvic organs. .

Many herbs are available and will be prescribed by the herbal practitioner according to specific needs. A good diet is essential, together with supplements of B complex, vitamin E, calcium and lecithin.

Agood tonic to take during the menopause is prepared by mixing equal quantities of hops, centaury, agrimony, wormwood and bog bean, adding 2oz (50g) of the well mixed herbs to 2 pints (1 litre) of cold water. This should be brought to the boil and simmered gently for fifteen minutes. Strain, take half a teacupful before meals daily.

Another useful remedy, which is relaxing to the nerves, relieving some of the nervous tension which can dominate, consists of equal amounts of raspberry leaves, lime blossom and pulsatilla herb. Mixed well, add one teaspoonful to a teacupful of boiling water, cover and infuse for five minutes.

Honey can be added to taste, or even milk and a little sugar.

The raspberry leaves will strengthen pelvic muscles; the other two herbs will have a cheering effect. Other remedies for depression are vervain and borage.

The discomforts which arise during and after the menopause are due to hormonal changes taking place at the time. The main female hormone, oestrogen is reduced, and so is progesterone, the hormone which mainly controls menstruation. Orthodox treatment offers. Hormone replacement therapy (HRT) which, it is claimed, will maintain normality and stave off the ageing process. Many doctors have their doubts about the treatment, although many women who have been on HRT for a number of years remain perfectly well. There is evidence to indicate a relationship between HRT and the increase in cancer of the endometrium (the inner wall of the uterus) and the breast. It is also linked with gall-bladder disease and high blood-pressure. Any woman who is having HRT should be under constant close observation by her doctor, so as to monitor her condition. There can be excessive weight gain, nausea, aggravation of varicose veins, tenderness of the breasts and the possibility of fibroid development in the uterus.

Herbal remedies which are not hormones themselves, but which encourage the body to produce its own hormones in the right balance, can be taken with complete safety.

One of the most useful of these is prepared from the plant vitex agnus castus. It is prescribed by the practitioner together with other herbal remedies which are not always easily available. It is the main ingredient in Gerard Agnus

Castus tablets and in the German Agnolyt remedy. Agnus castus has been found to regulate hormone imbalance before the menopause, when there can be over-production of oestrogen.

Other herbal tablets which can be of great help with menopausal symptoms are Napier's Menotabs and Roberts' Motherwort compound tablets. Many of the 'nerve' tablets or compounds available can be taken to reinforce these specific menopausal herbs with benefit and without any side-effects.

Diet during the menopause should include plenty of raw fresh salads and fruits, whole grains, adequate mixed proteins and must exclude processed and 'junk' foods.

Menstrual Disorders

Many remedies are available to treat menstrual disorders, whether the problem is painful, heavy, light or irregular periods. Infusions of wild yam, melilot, pulsatilla herb, balm or German chamomile can be taken to relieve pain at period times. One teaspoonful to teacupful of boiling water infused (covered) for ten minutes then strained, and taken in wineglassful doses three or four times daily is the method for anyone of them. Wild yam is useful for pain low in the abdomen, in the ovaries or womb; taken warm with a pinch of powdered ginger added it will give quick relief. Asmaller dose, a dessertspoonful, can be taken warm every two hours to relieve pain, but less often if the period is heavy. Melilot is the remedy for spasmodic, colicky pain, pain with a feeling of fullness and throbbing, especially if associated with a throbbing headache. Pulsatilla will help when nervous problems are dominant, when there are fears and dreads of calamity or melancholy and depression. It should be taken throughout the menstrual cycle when its influence on the nervous system and pelvic organs will gradually improve pain and irregularity. Balm, too, benefits the nervous system, is especially recommended for cramp-like pain during periods, can be taken up to six times daily at such times and two or three times daily between periods for its influence on headaches, insomnia, poor digestion and other nervous symptoms. German chamomile can be taken in a stronger infusion to relieve premenstrual migraine and pain during the period – 1 tablespoonful added to a cupful of boiling water, covered and left to infuse for an hour. It should be strained and sipped warm for quick relief,with a little lemon juice added.

Motherwort relieves irritability in pelvic nerves, tones up the uterine membrane, has a gentle strengthening action on the heart, and helps to regulate light periods. It can be taken in infusion and is also available in tablet form.

Napier's Motherwort and Rutin tablets will improve poor circulation; Roberts' Female Restorative tablets contain motherwort, gentian, uva ursi, valerian, pulsatilla and vervain, a comprehensive formula.

Premenstrual tension is the cause of much misery, irritability, tender breasts, headaches, bloated abdomen and other discomforts. Agnus castus tablets, Roberts'

Female Restorative tablets, or evening primrose capsules have been found to give much relief. An experiment, carried out on 300 women taking these capsules and specific vitamins, showed that an average of 76 per cent gained great relief and only two or three had no change at all in their PMT.

A change of diet during the week before a period is due can minimize the symptoms. A raw-food diet, in which there is very little salt has helped some women. A good diet generally can contribute to improvement in the periods, together with calcium, which soothes nerves, vitamin B complex which normalizes blood sugar, helps destroy excessive hormones and provides nutrition to the nerves, vitamin A to minimize irritability, lecithin which can be a tranquillizer and vitamin C to help eliminate body fluid.

No woman need suffer unnecessarily; the measures given above should be of great help. The herbal practitioner has many more remedies he can prescribe. Self-treatment should not be attempted for any abnormal symptoms, a diagnosis must be obtained.

Mental Fatigue

A wineglassful three times daily of sage tea, made by adding one teaspoonful of crushed dried leaves or six large fresh ones to 1/2 pint (0.25 litre) of boiling water, covering and leaving to cool, will help to clear the mind of fatigue, as will the same dose of either balm or rosemary. These are made in stronger infusions - one teaspoonful of herb to a teacupful of boiling water. Peppermint tea is refreshing to both mind and body, and should be infused for ten minutes to obtain its full potential. A little honey may be added to any of these tisanes. A little antispasmodic tincture rubbed well into the back of the neck and across the forehead, each morning and evening, can help when there is sustained mental work. Roberts' Avexan tablets, based on years of experience in practice, improve the ability to concentrate, containing avena (oats) reinforced in its action by prickly ash bark.

A brief change of occupation will relieve mental fatigue, either by spending a few minutes on physical exercises or work, or directing the attention to a different subject.

Migraine

The immediate and local cause of a migraine headache is swelling and inflammation of blood vessels in the head, but the causes which lead to this may be less easy to find.

Foods which contain certain amines - cheeses, chocolate, red wine, or sodium-nitrate-preserved meats in pies, etc., can trigger off an attack. Other foods will affect some sufferers but not others; migraine is very much an individual complaint. The cause should be found and dealt with, whether it be in the digestive system, due to nervous tension, constipation or disorders of the liver or kidneys, or psychosomatic. Migraine is often familial- about fifty per cent of sufferers have parents who also experience migraine - but that may only indicate dietetic and emotional family patterns. Migraine is found in the perfectionist, the person who must finish a task even though dropping with fatigue, who must have everything exactly right. Remedies will be of limited use unless this person becomes more relaxed and learns to look at life in a more philosophical way.

A number of herbs can give relief: an infusion of lavender flowers, leaves and stalks in teacupful doses, between meals, will be found to soothe the nervous system; if lavender oil is available, two drops can be taken on sugar and a little massaged gently on the painful temple and forehead. An infusion of vervain, lime blossom, rosemary or German chamomile will be relaxing and will help in the same way. Peppermint tea affords some relief to both headache and nausea. A few mint leaves moistened and bandaged gently on the forehead can work like magic easing the pain. A good combination to take regularly is equal quantities of motherwort, vervain, dandelion root chopped finely, centaury and wild carrot. Add 1 oz (25g) of the mixture to 1 pint (0.5 litre) of cold water, bring up to boiling point and simmer very gently for fifteen minutes.

Strain when cool. A wineglassful three times daily is an adequate dose. Feverfew should not be neglected, as it has been responsible for some remarkable cures. Certain properties were considered to be lost when the plant was heated, and the fresh leaf taken in a sandwich became popular. Weleda have produced tablets and liquids in homoeopathic form, which avoid the bitter taste, and Potter's have produced their own feverfew tablet.

Diet should avoid fried, fatty and dairy foods, should be semi-vegetarian and should include plenty of salads and fresh vegetables.

Multiple Sclerosis

Investigation has so far shown that evening primrose oil (available in capsule form) is the one herb which can help to counteract the damage to the myelin sheath covering of spinal nerves, the pathological cause of this disease.

Taken daily, combined with a gluten-free diet, the condition can usually at least be controlled.

Much research has been carried on into the dietetic background of MS, and a theory that the body's intolerance of gluten leads to the disease has been and is being studied.

Gluten is the protein in wheat and other grains.

Nausea

This unpleasant sensation is the body's way of indicating that something iswrong in the stomach or digestive system.

Food should not be taken at all until it has cleared.

Tisanes of chamomile, peppermint, mint or lime blossom will help, and should be taken three or four times daily.

Failing these, chewing some crystallized ginger might succeed. An infusion of tarragon herb is prepared by adding 1 oz (25g) to 2 pints (1 litre) of boiling water and allowing to infuse (covered) for ten minutes. A cupful, slightly warm, should allay the nausea. Antispasmodic tincture, taken in teaspoonful doses every hour or two, well diluted in warm sweetened water, will resolve the nausea in one way or another. Weleda's Melissa compound taken in water every hour will also relieve nausea. It includes the spices coriander, clove, nutmeg and cinnamon, which deal effectively with flatulence and stomach pains.

If nausea cannot be cleared by fasting and by these remedies, consult a practitioner.

Nervous Disorders

Various 'nervous' symptoms occur as the result of undue stress, or when the general health has been undermined by illness. Some of us inherit a nervous temperament, making us more sensitive to stresses and unhappiness.

Additionally, nervous symptoms may in some persons be an allergic response. Tension, irritability, disturbed sleep, palpitations and anxiety over trivia can make life more difficult for us and for those around us.

Many herbs are available to relax tension, to help the sufferer enjoy restful sleep and to improve digestion, thus ensuring better nutrition to the nervous system. Prompt treatment with herbal medicine can avoid the dreaded commitment to long-term tranquillizers and antidepressants.

Antispasmodic tincture, taken in warm sweetened water two or three times daily will make a good start to treatment. It contains valerian, a soothing remedy useful for the relief of irritability, and skull cap, a herb long-used as a tonic to the nervous system, relieving tension and spasmodic conditions. It can be reinforced by appropriate remedies taken as herbal teas twice daily or as required: vervain to lift feelings of depression and as a tonic through its influence on the liver; chamomile or balm for a 'nervous' stomach, nausea or poor appetite, or for a fluttering feeling in the stomach (antispasmodic tincture would help with all these too); an infusion of hops in a warm bedtime bath to promote a drowsiness conducive to sleep, especially if a cup of soothing herbal tea is sipped in bed afterwards.

Symington's 'Good Night herbal tea' contains valerian, lemon balm, peppermint, hops, yarrow, chamomile, and lavender flowers, and is a very soothing mixture. Weleda Malvae comp. herbal tisane contains lavender flowers, valerian root and blue mallow flowers, leading to peaceful relaxation.

A good combination as a general nerve tonic is equal quantities of valerian root, gentian root (both finely chopped), vervain, chamomile, catmint and skull cap. Mix the herbs well, add a teaspoonful to a teacupful of boiling water, cover and leave to infuse for ten minutes. Strain and drink before meals. A little honey may be added, in which case it would be better taken between meals.

Woodruff is a useful herb which benefits the nervous system. It can be taken two or three times daily to relax excessive nervous tension, for vertigo, neuralgia, and will ease the type of pain at period times which is caused by tension, and if taken at bedtime will help to give a good night's sleep.

The Bach flower remedies have been used with much success in treating nervous disorders: aspen for anxiety, olive for mental and physical tiredness, white chestnut for persistent unwanted thoughts and mustard or gentian for depression. These herbs, in homoeopathic dosage, can be taken with perfect safety and confidence.

There are many excellent preparations for nervous problems available from health food stores and from herbal suppliers. Such is the high standard of these that it would be impossible to single out any for recommendation. One would wish to recommend all.

The plan for treatment must include good nutrition, fresh air and exercise, adequate rest, and the deliberate cultivation of a positive attitude of mind. A whole food diet enriched with wheat germ, sunflower and sesame seeds, molasses, supplements of kelp, vitamin B complex and calcium tablets will enable the herbal remedies to be much more effective more quickly.

Nettle Rash

A skin rash, urticaria, which may be due to some allergen such as shellfish or penicillin, causes large smooth red wheals on the skin which appear quickly, itch severely and die down after two days. Giant urticaria produces very large swellings which can be painful. Avoid normal food, drink plenty of nettle tea and bathe the skin with the same infusion. Add a handful of fresh nettles, or 1 oz (25g) of dried ones, to 1pint (0.5 litres) of water, simmer gently for five minutes, take from the heat and leave to infuse for ten minutes. Add honey to the drink, but not to the lotion.

Echinacea or Blue Flag Root tablets or Roberts' Three-way skin treatment may be used. Occasional doses of antispasmodic tincture will ease the reaction via the nervous system. If the urticaria is recurrent and the food to which one is allergic cannot be discovered, seek the help of an herbal practitioner.

Nettle stings should be rubbed thoroughly with dock leaves, antispasmodic tincture or elderflower cream.

Neuritis and Neuralgia

Inflammation of the nerves can often result from injury, strain, deficiency of vitamin B or calcium, be caused by a virus or be due to inadequate alkaline elements in the diet.

The first remedy to consider is St John's Wort, taking the normal infusion of wineglassful doses three or four times daily. It has a sedative action and a locally analgesic action on nerve pains, especially sciatica and neuralgia. If oil can be made and kept ready for emergencies, this can be applied over the painful area several times daily. A handful of fresh St john's Wort herb placed in a glass jar, covered with good quality (first pressing) olive oil, with muslin to keep out dust, left to stand in the sun for six weeks, then strained through a fine cloth, will be a useful oil for neuralgia and neuritis. Keep in a cool place. Massage a little antispasmodic tincture, oil of lavender, Olbas oil, or a double-strength infusion of St John's Wort along the area of the pain. It may be possible to find a 'trigger' spot, a small area of intense tenderness and pain. If so, the antispasmodic tincture or oil of lavender should be massaged thoroughly into that. An infusion of melilot, or wood betony, taken three or four times daily, will reduce inflammation and thus relieve pain. The leaves or lotion of either can be applied as compresses over the pain. The fresh leaves of woodruff applied over neuralgic pain will quickly ease the intensity.

Roberts' Nerfood or Pulsatilla tablets, Gerard Valerian compound tablets and Heath & Heather's Nerve tablets each contain valerian and other herbal remedies to ease nerve pains and to promote a feeling of relaxation. Herbal sedative tablets can be taken with perfect safety, without causing drowsiness at the wrong time.

A combination of nerve and inflammation remedies, lotion or oil applied locally and a diet which accentuates green leafy vegetables, salads and adequate mixed protein will gradually but effectively overcome neuritis and neuralgia. If there is no improvement, consult a herbal practitioner.

Nightmares

Terrifying dreams can be the result of some disturbing experience in the past or be part of a nervous disorder. A tea of wood betony, one teaspoonful to a cupful of boiling water taken at bedtime, will help. Another effective remedy is chamomile tea, either alone or combined with balm in equal quantities, taken once or twice daily and also at bedtime; it will calm and relax the nervous system. If bad dreams are persistent, the Bach remedy, rock rose, will probably put an end to them.

Noises in the Ears (See Tinnitus)

Nosebleed

This can be quickly controlled by using nettles, either the juice from crushed leaves and stalks applied in the nostril on cotton wool, or simply a crushed leaf inserted as high as is comfortable. Don't forget to wear gloves when handling the nettles! A plug of cotton wool soaked in distilled witch-hazel, or tincture of St John's Wort if available, or the fresh crushed leaves of yarrow, herb Robert, cranes bill or golden rod. Keep the head back, not forward, to enable the blood to clot more easily.

Obesity

During recent years slimming diets have proliferated. The accumulation of extra body weight is most commonly due to consistent over-eating over many years, also due to hormonal changes, and to excessive intake of fluids and salt. One form of increased body weight, which is the least easy to control, is that which follows a hysterectomy.

Some herbal remedies can be used to improve metabolism, to eliminate excessive body fluid and to break down fatty deposits, and are used successfully when combined with a strict reduction of salt and all sugar and starchy foods. One day each week on small quantities of diluted fruit juice and either raw fruit (with the exception of bananas) or raw salads at mealtimes (no cheese, bread or any other food at all) will stimulate the metabolism and aid weight loss. The loss should be gradual.

An infusion of fennel seeds, 1 teaspoonful crushed seeds to a teacupful of boiling water, covered and left to cool, taken two or three times daily, or an infusion of white horehound 1 oz (25g) to 2 pints (1 litre) of boiling water) taken in wineglassful doses several times daily, the whole litre each day, would be helpful. Fucus or kelp tablets influence weight control through their action on the thyroid gland, but a practitioner must be consulted before taking them if there is, or has been, any thyroid problem.

The diet must be a comprehensive one, providing a good range of essentials: protein, minerals, vitamins, raw fresh foods. Too many enthusiastic slimmers have suffered from exhaustion because of an inadequate diet.

Osteomalacia

A painful condition in which the softening of bones occurs in later life, as a result of a diet deficient in minerals, or due to many years of digestive disorders and faulty assimilation.

A good balanced diet is essential, with plenty of sunshine to give the body vitamin D. Liver and gall-bladder remedies are applicable, and comfrey tea infused with a couple of bay leaves is useful to strengthen the bones and encourage calcification.

Osteoporosis

Thinning and weakening of the bone structure found in elderly persons is due to withdrawal of calcium from bone.

Hormonal changes at the menopause can lead to deprivation of calcium. Treatment consists of a nutritional diet which includes plenty of celery, parsley, green leafy vegetables, oats and other whole grains, vitamin D, vitamin C, and a wineglassful three times daily of comfrey and bay leaf tea. (One teaspoonful of comfrey leaves and 1bay leaf to a teacup of boiling water.)

Prevention of both conditions is by sound diet and plenty of exercise to maintain a good circulation.

Pain

The herbal practitioner does not use powerful pain-killers, but will seek causes and will select appropriate herbs to influence them and thus give relief. The first general remedy which springs to the mind is St John's Wort, effective for neuralgic pains. It was used by the Crusaders to ease and heal their wounds. If the fresh plant is heated gently in good olive oil, until almost crisp, it will produce a liniment useful for rheumatic pains, neuralgia and neuritis. The plant can also be infused in boiling water, allowed to cool to blood heat and applied as a warm compress, herb and liquid together. Comfrey leaf can be used in exactly the same way, and will very quickly ease the sharp pain of a sprain or fall. Lavender flowers and leaves prepared in oil, will relieve the pain of burns. Infused, a teaspoonful of flowers and leaves to a teacupful of boiling water, lavender will give relief from nervous headaches, taken in wineglassful doses. A poultice of crushed linseed will ease muscular pains, neuritis, painful boils, and period pains.

The crushed seeds should be mixed to a smooth paste with boiling water, spread on muslin and applied warm. It should be wrapped firmly in position and changed every twelve hours.

Amongst proprietary remedies, antispasmodic tincture will ease many types of pain. It may be taken in warm water for colic and stomach pains, for neuralgia, for headaches and may also be massaged over a painful area. Gerard Ligvites have relieved rheumatic pains, Heath & Heather's Backache tablets imply their use, and many others formulated as a result of long experience in herbal medicine are beneficial.

Palpitations

Palpitations, by which is meant consciousness of heartbeat and a more rapid beat, is most commonly due to nerves, dyspepsia, toxic stimulants such as tobacco, alcohol and coffee, or to over-exertion. It can also be a symptom of certain lung or heart conditions, anaemia, disorder of the thyroid gland or be caused by some drug treatment. It can occur during exhaustion or mild anaemia, following an illness. In such cases an infusion of motherwort herb in wineglassful doses, three or four times daily, will gently strengthen heart action. Add one teaspoonful to a teacupful of boiling water, cover and leave to infuse for ten minutes.

The herbal practitioner uses hawthorn for palpitations; an infusion of flowers and leaves (a teaspoonful to a cupful of boiling water) will have a sedative effect on heart action and on the circulation. Take it in wineglassful doses during the day, or half a cupful at bedtime. Balm, a gentle sedative, is another useful remedy for palpitations. Add 1 oz (25g) to a generous 1 pint (0.5 litres) of boiling water, cover and infuse for ten minutes. The dose is a wineglassful three times daily.

The cause of palpitations should be found and treated. If the above remedies have no effect, it is necessary to consult a practitioner.

Pharyngitis

An extension of a sore throat, cold or virus infection, pharyngitis should be treated as an infection.

Gargle with an infusion of sage (the normal infusion) every three or four hours. Add tincture of myrrh to the infusion, twenty drops to a teacupful. Drink a combination of sage and liquorice, a wineglassful every four hours. Add one peeled liquorice stick and 1oz (25g) of sage to 1 ½ pints (0.75 litre) of boiling water, simmer gently for two minutes, covered, leave to cool and strain. Wild indigo is valuable for its antibiotic properties, and lungwort is a useful remedy too. The normal infusion oflungwort taken in wineglassful doses, three or four times daily, should be adequate.

Phlebitis

Swelling, pain and stiffness in one area of the leg, usually the lower calf, can be an indication of inflammation of a vein. Rest in bed is essential for at least the first few days.

Distilled witch-hazel should be applied frequently, alternating with cold water compresses. Wring out soft cotton material, six or eight-fold thickness, in cold water and place firmly over the area. Replace each time it begins to feel warm. A useful tea can be made from a mixture of yarrow, witch-hazel leaves, comfrey root, broom tops, wild carrot and divers in equal quantities. One ounce (25g) of the mixture simmered gently in 1 pint (0.5 litre) of water, then strained, should be taken in wineglassful doses three or four times daily. Rutin tablets should be taken to strengthen the blood vessels.

There will be risk of a thrombus (blood dot) forming and grave dangers of it breaking off and passing in the circulation to the heart or lungs. For this reason self treatment is inadequate and a practitioner must be consulted.

Piles *(see* Haemorrhoids)

Pleurisy

This acute inflammation of the membrane covering the lungs makes every breath intensely painful. The primary remedy, used by the American Indians, is pleurisy root. It can be used alone, the chopped root simmered gently for ten minutes, or combined with hyssop, marshmallow root and liquorice root. Take equal quantities of these herbs, add 2oz (50g) to 2 pints (I litre) of cold water, bring to the boil and simmer gently for ten minutes. Leave to cool slightly, strain and take a wineglassful hot every two hours.

This will induce perspiration and will ease the pain by reducing inflammation.

Use *2 oz* (50g) each of pleurisy root, marshmallow root, liquorice root and slippery elm bark to 3 pints (1.5 litres) of boiling water, simmered down to 1pint (0.5 litre).

The dose of this is a half-teaspoonful dose every half-hour.

The painful area should be rubbed with a warming liniment and covered immediately with warm flannel. It is essential to rest in bed, to keep warm and to have no food whatsoever until the symptoms have eased and the temperature is normal. It would be wise to seek the advice of a practitioner, especially if the symptoms do not improve with treatment.

Polypus

Best treated by a practitioner. If obtainable, tincture of blood root can be used to paint nasal polypi - it is eventually effective but other treatment is necessary in conjunction.

Pregnancy and Childbirth

Two remedies are paramount for the pregnant woman: raspberry leaves and chamomile flowers. The raspberry leaves should be taken after the third month until the birth, in wineglassful doses, three times daily, *1 oz* (25g) to 1pint (0.5 litre) of boiling water, infused for ten minutes then strained. Raspberry leaf is astringent and tonic, will strengthen uterine and pelvic muscles, act to prevent miscarriage and will help to make the birth easier. Taken warm, in teacupful doses with a pinch of composition powder or a teaspoonful of the essence added, raspberry leaves will facilitate labour and should be taken every hour at that time. They can also be continued after the birth to tone and strengthen the pelvic tissues. If difficulties arise with the afterbirth, an infusion of marshmallow leaves will help release it. Add *1 oz* (25g) to 1pint (0.5 litre) of boiling water, cover and infuse for ten minutes.

Chamomile flowers can be taken in teacupful doses, as required, to alleviate morning sickness, cramps, nerve pains or indigestion. Toxaemia during pregnancy is often due to faulty diet. A good lacto-vegetarian diet with lots of salads, green vegetables and with supplements of vitamin B complex and kelp, should help prevent it from occurring. Raspberry leaves have blood-cleansing properties, and should also help. Lime blossom tea can be taken for raised blood-pressure.

Prolapse

Prolapse of the womb requires professional attention; a practitioner experienced in this will advise on exercises to help, will probably be able to return the womb to its normal position if it is not too badly prolapsed, and will help in other ways. Raspberry leaf tea is essential, a wineglassful three times daily. The infusion, strained through fine cloth or a paper coffee filter and warmed to blood heat, can be used as a douche. A combination of motherwort, raspberry leaves and tansy - equal quantities mixed well and added to cold water in the normal quantity will be very useful in improving the muscle-tone. Add 1 oz (25g) to 1pint (0.5 litre) of water, bring to the boil and simmer gently for ten minutes. This should be taken in half-cupful doses after each meal. Deep abdominal breathing, as used in some yoga exercises, should be avoided.

Neither surgery, which shortens the ligaments holding the womb in position, nor a ring to hold the womb up, are recommended unless totally unavoidable.

Prostate Gland

The prostate gland surrounds the commencement of the male urethra. It is about the size of a chestnut and can become congested, inflamed and enlarged, causing pain, frequent and urgent passing of urine, sometimes burning.

It may be permanently enlarged in the older man, causing no pain but affecting the flow of urine. Constipation aggravates the problem and should be avoided.

A good diet rich in fresh raw salads and vegetables, whole-wheat bread, and added sunflower seeds and zinc tablets (which help the body to produce hormones needed by the gland) is necessary as a means of maintaining a healthy prostate. A vegetarian diet is more health-giving sugar, salt, milk, alcohol, tea and coffee should all be kept to the minimum.

The herbal practitioner uses a number of remedies to deal with both acute and chronic prostate troubles. A good combination is 1oz (25g) each of horse tail, couch grass and hydrangea - with ½ oz (12.5g) of juniper berries. Add half the quantity to 2 pints (1 litre) of water bring to the boil and simmer gently for five minutes. Remove from heat and strain when cool. The dose is a wineglassful three times daily. Roberts' Black Willow compound tablets, the result of many years of experience in practice, are very good indeed for prostatic disorders.

Acute and painful prostatic problems must be attended to by a practitioner.

Pruritis

The rash and intense itching affecting either vaginal or anal areas may be of nervous origin. If it is mostly around the anus and worse at bedtime, it could be caused by threadworms. Pruritis often occurs in later life and may be due to dietary deficiencies.

Alotion made from elderflowers should be applied freely to relieve itching and herbal remedies for the blood and nerves should be taken daily.

Roberts' pruritis ointment or Weleda Sambucus compound are both well-tried and successful remedies for the condition. If there is no improvement after trying these remedies for two or three weeks, a practitioner must be consulted, as persistent pruritis can be a symptom of more serious disorders.

Psoriasis

A chronic, hereditary recurrent skin disease, many cases of which respond to herbal medicine. Persistence with treatment is necessary. A herbal tea consisting of equal quantities of divers, burdock root, dandelion root, yellow dock root and red dover flowers, prepared as a decoction and taken in wineglassful doses, three times daily, will provide a foundation treatment, dealing with impurities in the blood-stream, improving liver function and elimination via the kidneys. Echinacea tablets taken twice daily will reinforce the action.

A number of prepared remedies are available and will be found to contain blue flag root, nettles, echinacea and sarsaparilla in varying quantities, as well as the herbs given above. Heath & Heather's Blood Purifying mixture and Potter's Skin Clear tablets are amongst those which can be obtained from the health food stores. Roberts' Three Way skin treatment for psoriasis, Gerard Blue Flag tablets or Red Clover, chaparral and ginseng tablets may be taken with confidence.

Herbal teas of balm, nettle or raspberry leaf, taken in wineglassful doses, three times daily, may also be used as a lotion, prepared as a normal infusion. Each psoriasis sufferer is different: the sum total of heredity, glandular imbalance, stresses, or a lifetime diet which may have led to deficiency of vitamins and minerals. No single course of treatment is a remedy for all psoriasis; it may be necessary to find the right combination to suit the individual.

Applications to the skin are not the herbalist's primary approach but can be helpful. Yarrow has been found to help clear psoriasis - taken twice-weekly in a warm bath it promotes perspiration and clears impurities through the pores. The herbs are infused for fifteen minutes, 1 oz (25g) to 1 pint (0.5 litre), the liquid added to the bath water and the herbs in a muslin bag used as a compress and to scrub the patches. Chickweed ointment may be applied afterwards, or Napier's Poke Root ointment.

A vegetarian diet is preferable, one rich in green salads, watercress, green leafy vegetables, nettles cooked as spinach, celery, carrots (raw carrots should be eaten every day), all fresh raw fruits except gooseberries, plums and rhubarb, whole-wheat bread, nuts, pulses (lentils, peas, beans), sunflower seeds, millet, eggs, some cheese and very little milk. Some psoriasis sufferers may need to avoid milk and dairy products. Supplement the diet with vitamin B complex, dolomite tablets and vitamin C (500mg) daily.

The foods to be strictly avoided are sugar, white flour products, salt, processed and 'convenience' foods.

Quinsy

This painful malady produces small abscesses on or near the tonsil. It should be treated in the same way as tonsillitis, by fasting, gargling with herbal infusions, cold compresses around the throat and herbal remedies taken internally.

Make a normal infusion of sage leaves and divide equally when cool. To one portion add an equal quantity of infusion of hyssop and some tincture of myrrh (10 drops to a teacupful) and use this as a gargle, several times daily. To the other portion add an infusion of one teaspoonful of thyme herb in a teacupful of boiling water, covered and infused for five minutes, and either twenty drops of tincture of wild indigo, or a tablespoonful of composition essence. Take two tablespoonfuls of this mixture four times daily. In addition, take garlic oil capsules at bedtime. Echinacea tablets would help to eliminate the poisons.

See also Tonsillitis.

Rheumatism

The term rheumatism covers a variety of disorders in which inflammation in muscles and soft tissues causes swelling, pain and stiffness, and can ultimately lead to degenerative changes. In addition to the localized symptoms, the general health can be affected.

Tiredness and weight loss are early signs; ungainly walking and distorted joints can be the culmination of many years' suffering. Causes are many, or unknown. Faulty nutrition, trauma, stress, and negative emotions such as chronic resentment or perfectionism may be responsible.

Many herbs are used in the treatment of rheumatism; the herbal practitioner prepares his formula according to the individual needs of the patient, after a careful assessment of the patient's health and specific type of rheumatism and adjusts the medication as treatment progresses.

Celery is one of the finest anti-rheumatic remedies. It can be included in dispensed medicine, the stalks can be eaten daily in salad, the powdered seed is a good substitute for salt and a tea can be made from the seeds. Celery has antiseptic properties, helps relieve the pain of rheumatism and, as a bonus, aids digestion and appetite and is sedative to the nervous system. The tea is made by adding one teaspoonful of the crushed seeds to a teacupful of boiling water; it should be covered and left to cool, then strained and the one teacupful taken (in parts) at intervals during the day. A good combination of herbs is equal quantities of celery seed (crushed), bog bean, yarrow, yellow dock root and red clover, mixed well together, and 2 oz (50g) of the mixture added to 2 pints (1 litre) of boiling water and simmered gently for fifteen minutes, left to cool (still covered) and half a teacupful taken before meals. Sage is reputed to dissolve uric acid, clivers and gravel root both help to eliminate it through the kidneys.

The pain of rheumatism can be relieved, in many instances, by herbal compresses. Some of the herbs can be taken internally at the same time, providing a double treatment. An infusion of chamomile flowers (Matricaria, the German variety) will be gently sedative and anti inflammatory.

It may be taken in wineglassful doses and the flowers applied as a moist poultice over the painful joint - cool if the joint is hot and inflamed, otherwise warm. Wood betony can be used in the same way for chronic rheumatism. Meadowsweet is included in most formulae for its antacid properties, a fine antidote for uric acid which deposits in crystal form in the joints. The flowers are infused, covered for ten minutes in water which is just under boiling point. The dose is a teacupful three times daily, before breakfast, mid-afternoon and at bedtime. The flowers applied as a poultice around a joint will relieve the pain. The tea should be taken regularly for a few weeks.

Effective as these remedies are, there are times when it is much more convenient to have ready-prepared mixtures.

There are many from which to choose from health food stores. Celery seeds are available, also Potter's Nine Rubbing Oils - a long-established liniment for the relief of rheumatic pains, which can be used in conjunction with their rheumatic herbs and tablets. Heath & Heather have a number of remedies for rheumatic pain, in powder, tablet or liquid form and Weleda have produced a very good massage balm. Practitioners have, of course, prepared their own compounds from many years' experience in practice, and can supply details.

Rickets

This condition was thought to have been eliminated in the western world but occasionally cases are being seen again. A deficiency of vitamin D and sunlight, coupled with poor nutrition, disturbs the normal growth and calcification of bones, leading to muscular pain and bending of weight bearing bones.

A good diet of protein, fresh vegetables, fruits and whole grains is necessary. Oats, which contain minerals necessary in bone building, should form a high proportion of cereals in the form of porridge and muesli and be used in baking. Iceland moss should be given daily, a teaspoonful to a cupful of hot water, or milk and water, sweetened with molasses or honey to taste and a sprinkle of grated nutmeg, can be taken as a hot drink, or left to cool and eaten as a nutritious jelly. Parsley, for its vitamin and mineral content, should also be taken regularly.

Ringworm

An unpleasant skin disease caused by a fungus, it should be treated with strict hygiene, local applications, garlic capsules each night and herbal medicine.

A lotion can be made by simmering a handful of fresh elder leaves (washed) in enough water to cover them, with two crushed garlic cloves and a small handful of herb robert, very gently for three minutes. Remove from heat and leave to cool. Soak a piece of lint or cotton wool in the liquid and bathe the patches two or three times daily.

Crushed burdock leaves may also be used as a poultice.

Combine equal quantities of yarrow, sage, thyme and mint, add a teaspoonful of the mixture to a teacupful of boiling water, cover and leave to cool. Meanwhile, add 1 oz (25g) of crushed burdock root to 1 pint (0.5 litres) of cold water, bring to the boil and simmer gently for fifteen minutes. Leave to cool and do not strain until using it.

Take a cupful of each - the burdock decoction and the yarrow mixture - mix them and drink at intervals during the day.

Massaging the ringworm patches with castor oil has been found effective in some cases.

Rupture (See Hernia)

Sciatica

Pain in the sciatic nerve, which runs down (he back of the leg to the knee, arises from pressure in the lower spine, from inflammation of the nerve itself or from some back strain or injury, in which case treatment by an osteopath will help.

Hot fomentations of St John's Wort can, in many cases, give quick relief. Make the normal infusion, allow it to stand for ten minutes, take a wineglassful of the liquid three times daily and apply the hot liquid and herb as a compress, taking care not to scald the skin. Encase the herb in fine cotton fabric or muslin. Rubbing with any of the herbal oils or creams which contain thyme, cajeput, wintergreen, etc., will help, in conjunction with herbal remedies such as Roberts' Sciatic tablets, Potter's Sciargo tablets, or Heath & Heather's Rheumatism, Sciatica and Lumbago mixture. Warmth, rest in a firm bed and warm baths containing nettles, will speed recovery.

Sea-Sickness (See Travel-Sickness)

Shingles

Shingles (Herpes Zoster) is an inflammatory skin eruption with much pain, burning and some itching, arising from the chickenpox virus, either previously dormant in the body or a recent contact, and often related to a lowered standard of vitality. The pain is felt two days to two weeks before the rash appears and, especially with older people, may linger for some months. The rash heals in one to three weeks. It appears in clusters, unilaterally.

Nerve remedies must be taken abundantly, rest and relaxation must be adequate, a good diet followed to supplement action of the herbal remedies, and vitamin B complex taken daily. Antispasmodic tincture should be started immediately, a half-teaspoonful dose in warm water three times daily, and the tincture painted several times daily onto the rash. St John's Wort is valuable in this condition, both as a tea and as a lotion. The tincture may be painted onto the rash daily. A lotion prepared from equal quantities of St John's Wort flowers and chamomile flowers, infused as in the normal way, will ease the pain.

Make it double strength if it is not effective enough.

Vitamin E has been found very helpful, both taken internally (starting at 300IU daily, increased only if there is no high blood-pressure) and the oil from the capsules applied twice daily.

Shock

The body's reaction to sudden trauma, an accident, serious burn, scald, or extremely distressing news.

Two herbal remedies can be used with absolute confidence and safety in all cases of shock: antispasmodic tincture, given in half-teaspoonful doses, in warm sweetened water, every fifteen minutes or half-hour and

Dr Bach's Rescue Remedy, one to three drops on the tongue or lips every few minutes. Sweetened peppermint tea is also good as a remedy to counteract shock. If nothing else is available, a teaspoonful of honey either swallowed slowly, or-taken in some warm water, will be useful. It is essential to keep warm, by wrapping or covering with blankets, rugs, coats or other clothing and by giving warm drinks.

Sinusitis

This is usually caused by the spread of infection from a cold or influenza, or from nasal catarrh. Chronic sinusitis produces headache across the forehead, acute pain in the face when out of doors in a cold wind, and periodic bouts of sneezing and blocked nasal passages.

Eyebright herb is excellent for sinus problems. Taken in wineglassful doses three times daily, it will help disperse catarrh and soothe inflamed mucous membranes. Elderflowers help too; if taken hot they will encourage catarrh to flow. A combination of equal quantities of yarrow, white horehound, peppermint and wild indigo, prepared as a normal infusion and taken in wineglassful doses three or four times daily, with the bedtime dose taken hot, will work wonders. Inhalations will improve the condition. Use eucalyptus oil, if available or an infusion of the leaves, or Olbas oil in a little hot water. Garlic oil capsules at bedtime will provide useful antiseptic action.

Diet and general health must be looked after. Avoid dairy products completely, have plenty of fresh vegetables (greens and onions in abundance) and salads every day.

Skin Problems

Skin problems are numerous, but so are the herbal remedies for them. The herbal practitioner will seek the causes and will select appropriate herbs, preferring to deal with a skin condition from within rather than only prescribing ointments or lotions. There is no single cause, no simple remedy. A skin eruption can be due to a faulty diet, or may arise as an allergic reaction to drug treatment or to a certain food. Many people are sensitive to the proteins in wheat, eggs and milk. Nutritional deficiencies, especially a lack of adequate vitamin A, C and various B vitamins, and faulty utilization of fats in the diet, have led to skin problems.

There may be malfunction of the liver and kidneys, putting greater burden on the skin as a means of elimination.

Indigestion can lead to increased production of toxins, also burdening the skin if the diet is excessive in refined carbohydrates; chronic constipation will also contribute.

Burdock root and yellow dock root are amongst the most widely used and valuable remedies for skin conditions, together with fumitory, sarsaparilla, chickweed, clivers and meadowsweet. They are included in the prepared remedies available. Heath & Heather use fumitory and burdock as the main ingredients in their Blood Purifying tablets. Abbott's Sassafras herbs are excellent for a wide range of skin conditions; Napier's Alterative tablets are helpful in treating irritative skin conditions, while Gerard tablets and Roberts' skin remedies are each founded on a practitioner's experience in practice. Echinacea tablets will reinforce whichever remedies are used.

A combination of burdock root and yellow dock root in equal quantities, *1 oz* (25g) to 1 1/2 pints (0.75 litre) of water, simmered gently down to 1 pint (0.5 litre) and taken in wineglassful doses, three or four times daily, will be effective for simple skin eruptions. A lotion made from elderflowers, *1 oz* (25g) to 1pint (0.5 litre) of boiling water, left to cool then strained through a fine cloth, will relieve itching, as will an infusion of marigold flowers, either *1 oz* (25g) of the whole flower head to 1pint (0.5 litre) of boiling water, or two teaspoonfuls of the petals to a cupful of boiling water. In either case, cover and infuse for fifteen minutes.

Strain and use as a lotion for an oily skin. An infusion of red clover flowers, the normal infusion, may be taken in wineglassful doses, before meals, and applied as a lotion to moist skin eruptions. Elderflower cream or ointment will be found to soothe many types of skin rashes and irritations.

Diet must of course be adjusted to eliminate sugar, white flour products, and rich and fatty foods. Vitamin supplements may need to be taken. Lecithin taken either in tablet or granule form will control metabolism of fat and cholesterol in the body, and this alone may affect a cure in some cases. Alkaline foods must form the major part of the diet - green leafy vegetables, salads and fruits.

Any persistent skin eruptions which do not respond to any of the herbal or dietary remedies given above must have professional attention.

Sprains

Apply something to the sprained joint as swiftly as possible to counteract the swelling and inflammation. A cold water compress will be effective as a first measure. What is used next depends on what is available: distilled witch-hazel, used full strength; tincture of arnica, diluted by adding one teaspoonful to a half-teacupful of cold water; an infusion of comfrey leaves, plantain leaves or St John's Wort herb. These herbs, if fresh leaves can be obtained, can be applied directly over the painful area and bandaged in place. They should be bruised first, and comfrey leaves, because of the rough hairy under surface, should be encased in fine cotton material. The comfrey leaves may also be softened first in hot water and the bandage moistened in the liquid. A firm bandage around the joint, not so tight as to impede circulation, kept moist with the chosen application, will quickly reduce inflammation and encourage the joint tissues to return to normal.

Stomach Disorders

A nervous disposition may be the cause of many recurrent stomach upsets. Liver or gall-bladder disorders will also contribute. The diet will probably need to be adjusted. A skilful practitioner will be able to assess the major problems and deal with them.

Slippery elm is a superb remedy, either as a drink or taken in tablet form, two tablets after meals. It contains mucilage, is soothing and healing, and the ingredients combined with it in tablet form will aid digestion. Taken as a drink between meals it will be nutritious as well as soothing.

There are a number of prepared remedies available from health food stores. The Weleda Carminative tisane will ease indigestion and relieve flatulence; both Potter's and

Heath & Heather's indigestion remedies are excellent. See also advice given under Digestive Disorders; Flatulence and Gastritis.

If the symptoms do not respond to the remedies and a change in diet has no effect, or if pain is persistent and there is weight loss, a practitioner must be consulted.

Stress

According to Dr Hans Selye, who has made a specific study of the effects of stress on the body, we cannot avoid stress as long as we live, but we C!1nlearn a great deal about how to keep its damaging side-effects to a minimum. Acertain amount of stress is necessary to stimulate our latent powers.

Herbal teas which can help minimize the results of overwhelming stress are chamomile, limeblossom, wood betony, balm, lavender, skull cap, valerian and melilot. An infusion of any, taken in wineglassful doses, three or four times daily, will relax the whole system. In addition, antispasmodic tincture taken occasionally or regularly, and

Dr Bach's Rescue Remedy available to take when the stresses become unbearable, will gradually show benefit.

If going through a period of unavoidable stresses, take any of the herbal teas three times daily, with a larger dose at bedtime, and a teaspoonful of antispasmodic tincture in warm water during the day when feeling tired.

Eat light, easily-digested meals, trying to avoid nibbling between meals, something many of us do for comfort. If sleep is disturbed have a hops bath at bedtime and take Passiflora or Quiet Life tablets.

See also Insomnia and Nervous Disorders.

Strokes

The remarks under the heading 'Thrombosis' are applicable. Treatment must be directed to improvement following the stroke and to preventing recurrence.

Wood betony is a good remedy to take as soon as possible after a stroke has occurred - one of the finest remedies for many head and brain conditions, neuralgia, headaches and others. A wineglassful of the normal infusion three times daily will go towards restoring normal function, as far as this is possible. Antispasmodic tincture should be rubbed well into the back of the neck right up to the base of the skull, as this will improve both nerve supply and circulation. Yarrow tea should be taken for its antithrombotic properties - a wine glassful two or three times daily. The herb marigold, 'herb of the sun', has been long esteemed for its benefits to blood vessels and could be useful following a stroke to help strengthen them: a teacupful daily, prepared by adding two teaspoonfuls of the petals to a cupful of hot water, covering and leaving to infuse for ten minutes. It could be combined with a half teaspoonful of lime blossom and will additionally be sedative and relaxing. Diet and intake of important substances, such as lecithin and vitamin E, as under 'Thrombosis' should be followed strictly.

Smoking, alcohol and coffee must be avoided.

Sunburn

Strong sun dries the skin's natural oils and the skin should be protected before exposing it. Sunbathe for short periods at first, increasing the length of time each day. A simple mixture of olive oil and cider vinegar, will prevent burning and will keep the skin moist. This should be applied before sunbathing, but under really powerful sunshine a lotion which filters the sun's rays would be a better choice.

Sesame oil could be incorporated in a lotion, as it absorbs the ultraviolet rays. Apply protective cream to lips and nose to prevent unsightly and painful sores and blistering.

If the skin has been burned, olive oil and cider vinegar, a greater amount of the vinegar, or a cool infusion of elderflowers, nettles or chamomile flowers, applied liberally will be soothing. Dab the whole area frequently to reduce the heat, sponge the whole body if necessary, drink plenty of cold water, sipping it rather than gulping it down. If available, comfrey oil, elder leaf oil, or St John's wort oil will quickly ease pain and lower the skin temperature.

Sunstroke
Rest in a cool shaded room, sponge the body all over with cold water or cool herbal infusions, and apply cold compresses to the most affected areas, replacing them as soon as they feel warm. Do not give any alcohol or stimulants. Treat for shock giving Rescue Remedy, Antispasmodic tincture, lavender tea (which can also be used to sponge the skin because of its sedative effect on the nerves), or peppermint tea. Wood betony tea would be helpful if there is a severe headache or some delirium. If the temperature does not return to normal with these measures get medical help.

Swellings
Treatment for any swelling depends on the type of swelling and its cause. It would be wise to have it examined by a practitioner.

An acute swelling, caused by an injury, will respond to a cold compress of witch-hazel, elderflower lotion or an infusion of nettles. Honey spread on cotton or linen fabric and fastened over the area will also ease discomfort and reduce the swelling.

Teething

Mix a little tincture of myrrh with honey to make a palatable paste and massage this gently on the gums with a cotton bud. Alternate this with encouraging the infant to suck and chew a stick of marshmallow root. Give two teaspoonfuls of chamomile tea, two or three times daily, in milk or sweetened water.

Tension

Many of the herbs recommended for nervous disorders will be found to ease tension, but, as always, the cause should be found and dealt with. Alack of calcium can lead to tension, nerve irritability and a feeling of twitchiness in the limbs. Deficiency of B vitamins may also contribute to tension. Stress, emotional problems and conflicts at work or at home are other causes.

Herbal teas taken regularly, together with a good diet, adequate healthy exercise, deep breathing and enough sleep should lead to a more relaxed state.

Valerian is a good remedy for tension; it contains silica and other minerals, and valerianic acid is antispasmodic and has a soothing, tranquillizing effect on the nervous system. Not pleasant in taste, it may be taken in tablet form and is one of the main constituents of many nerve remedies.

A favourable combination is valerian, skull cap and passiflora.

It is one of the ingredients of antispasmodic tincture.

Only small doses of valerian are needed; massive doses can cause headaches.

Throat

A gargle of sage, or equal quantities of sage and elderflower, or an infusion of blackberry leaves, can be used for a sore throat in the early stages of a cold or infection. Sage has antiseptic qualities, elderflowers reduce inflammation and temperature, and blackberry leaves are astringent and cooling. Another fine gargle is prepared by adding 1 oz (25g) of crushed bistort root to 1 pint (0.5 litre) of cold water, bringing to the boil slowly. Remove from heat when at boiling point and leave to infuse for fifteen minutes. A soothing and pleasant-tasting gargle is made from liquorice sticks. Peel the sticks and add 2 oz (50g) to 2 pints (1 litre) of cold water. Bring to the boil, simmer gently for ten minutes and strain when cool. Take a wine glassful three or four times daily and gargle several times each day. Do not forget that liquorice is slightly laxative.

Blackcurrant tea, for children's' sore throats, is a pleasant drink. It can be made from fresh or frozen unsweetened blackcurrants, a teaspoonful to a teacupful of boiling water, the berries mashed thoroughly. A teaspoonful of blackcurrant jam or jelly (preferably home-made) could be added, or a little honey.

See also Quinsy and Tonsillitis.

Thrombosis

A dangerous condition which must be treated by a practitioner.

The approach must be to prevent the thrombus (blood clot) from breaking away and passing in the bloodstream to block a blood vessel, and secondly to improve the quality of the blood by diet and herbal remedies to prevent recurrence. If a thrombus develops in a leg vein, the herbal practitioner will apply a warm poultice of slippery elm or some stimulating poultice of his own formula, advising that it should be changed every twelve hours.

Garlic has a powerful effect in reducing blood cholesterol and should be taken daily, either eaten in food or taken as deodorized oil capsules. Yarrow herb has been discovered to have anti-thrombotic properties; a wineglassful of the normal infusion, two or three times daily for several months, will improve the quality of the blood. Both nettle and hawthorn strengthen blood vessels and reduce deposits on vessel walls.

Animal fats must be replaced by vegetable oils high in lecithin. Soya, safflower and sunflower (in that order) are the highest. Lecithin can be taken in granular or tablet form, for the purpose of breaking down fats and emulsifying them, and reducing cholesterol deposits in blood vessels. The risk of thrombosis is then reduced. Vitamin E has been discovered to reduce clotting of blood in its early stages and to strengthen cell membranes of blood cells, thus also being a useful preventive measure. Plenty of salads and green leafy vegetables should be included in the diet, which would advisedly be vegetarian.

Tinnitus

There are several causes of noises in the ears: catarrh, fatigue, anxiety, anaemia, raised blood-pressure, to name a few. Garlic taken regularly has been effective in some cases, its antiseptic properties helping to clear catarrh. It can, of course, also help lower blood-pressure. A cupful of balm tea taken once or twice daily could be of some benefit.

A herbal practitioner would endeavour to find the cause and would have some specific remedies.

Tonsillitis

When the first signs of tonsillitis appear, take no food, have plenty of fresh lemon juice and honey in hot water, drink herbal teas several times daily and gargle every hour. Rest in bed and warmth will lead to a quicker recovery.

Combine ½ oz (12.5g) each of agrimony herb and raspberry leaves; add to 2 pints (1 litre) of boiling water, cover and leave to infuse for fifteen minutes. Strain and take a wineglassful four times daily. Take three drops of tincture of wild indigo in a little water alternately with this tea. If the tonsillitis is very severe take the herbal remedies in alternation with a vitamin C tablet and the biochemic tissue salt Ferr. phos., taking a dose every half-hour. An infusion of marshmallow leaves and flowers in wineglassful doses, four or five times daily, will soothe the throat. A few drops of wild indigo may be added for its anti-bacterial properties. Painting the tonsils is very effective, many practitioners have their own special throat oil; eucalyptus oil is a fine antiseptic for this purpose. Use a soft camel-hair brush. Special throat brushes may be available from some chemists.

If tonsillitis recurs frequently, avoid dairy products, change to a diet high in raw fruits, salads and vegetables, eat lots of blackberries in season. The blackberry has a tonic and astringent effect on mucous membrane, and its use in healing inflammation in the mouth has been known for centuries. An infusion of the leaves, dried preferably, will make a useful astringent gargle.

Consult a herbal practitioner if recurrent tonsillitis does not improve. Do not resort to surgery. The tonsils are part of the body's defence system and the first to give warning of infection.

Chronic tonsillitis can be overcome by persisting with the right, health-giving treatment.

Toothache

Obviously, dental treatment is necessary to deal with the cause of toothache, but to obtain relief apply oil of cloves.

If there is a cavity in the aching tooth a small plug of cotton wool soaked in the oil will give quick relief. If the tooth is intact paint the oil on the gums. Chewing fresh plantain leaves is another good remedy, as is a strong infusion of flowers and leaves of the common mallow. Chewing the infused flowers will be even more effective. The juice from a grated raw onion soaked onto a plug of cotton wool and applied to the tooth will be soothing.

Good dental health depends on a good diet and regular visits to the dentist. Chew a few borage leaves if courage is needed!

Travel Sickness

The irregular movements, rapid acceleration and deceleration, and altitude changes experienced in various forms of travel, disturb the mechanism of the middle ear, leading to nausea and the other unpleasant symptoms of travel sickness. The sight of swiftly-passing landscape can have a similar effect when travelling by car or train.

Nervousness or nervous anticipation of the journey serve to compound the problem.

Avoid rich foods before a journey, having only simple food which is normally easily digested. Ginger has been found to be one of the most successful remedies, eaten in either preserved or crystallized form, before or during the journey. If tincture of ginger is available, two or three drops to a tablespoonful of water can be carried in a small bottle to be sipped from time to time. Chamomile tea can help, as it is useful for allaying nausea. Antispasmodic tincture also gives relief, diluted before the journey, one teaspoonful to a small teacupful of slightly sweetened water. Both these remedies can be prepared before setting off.

Children's' travel sickness can be partly due to nerves but frequently due to the mixture of foods given before and during a journey to pacify the child. An apple or pear, a few grapes or a peeled carrot could be given to replace sweets, crisps, ice-cream and chocolate, and sparkling bottled spring water or diluted fruit juices given to quench thirst. Games which occupy the child in looking downwards and inside the vehicle, instead of at the passing scenery, may prevent the visual type of travel sickness from developing.

Fresh air when possible, or good ventilation, often allays nausea.

Tubercular Infection
Professional treatment must be sought, but this can be reinforced by good diet, adequate rest and fresh air, the avoidance of smoking and relief from anxiety.

Herbal teas can be taken which will not interfere with whatever treatment is being undertaken. Primary amongst these is comfrey root; chop 4 oz (100g) of root, add to 2 pints (1 litre) of tepid water, cover and leave to stand for four hours. Take a teacupful of these three or four times daily. The normal infusion of the leaves can also be taken before meals. Comfrey contains allantoin, a substance which promotes healing. The herb has been used for centuries for all lung disorders, including tuberculosis, to aid in healing of fractured bones, to reduce swelling and inflammation in strained muscles and to strengthen the muscles, as well as to heal sores and ulcers. The leaf is used externally and can also be taken as tea, but the root has a more powerful effect for lung conditions. It can be taken in the dose given above for long periods of time with perfect safety.

Hyssop is another valuable herb. The normal infusion is taken in two-tablespoonful doses before meals, a little honey added. Hyssop is an expectorant, and helps clear catarrh and mucus from the lungs.

Ulcers

Ulceration is the breakdown of surface tissues. There are herbs rich in mucilage and other soothing constituents; astringents which will help the tissues knit together and herbal antiseptics to cleanse. The herbal practitioner will select from these as the individual patient needs.

Mouth ulcers, usually pointing to hyperacidity, can be cleared by application several times daily of tincture of myrrh, either full strength (it will smart) or diluted. In the dilution of one teaspoonful to a cupful of warm water it can be used as a mouthwash. An infusion of bistort root or blackberry leaves (one teaspoonful of either to a teacupful of boiling water) used as a mouthwash will clear the ulcers.

Leg ulcers need professional attention. Poultices of comfrey leaf, slippery elm, chickweed, yarrow or marigold flowers can help, but must be supplemented by taking blood purifiers such as echinacea tablets (see also Blood Disorders and Varicose Veins). Napier's calendula ointment has been found helpful;

comfrey ointment will heal. It is important to cleanse the body, not merely to close up an outlet for poisons.

Stomach ulcers also need to be under the care of a herbal practitioner. Benefit can be obtained from slippery elm, golden seal (available in tablet form) papaya tablets, nerve remedies and possibly a change of life-style. (See Duodenal Ulcer.)

Urinary Disorders

A heading which could cover a multitude of problems, some dealt with separately under Cystitis; Enuresis; and Kidney Disorders, page 90. It would be wise to have a diagnosis and professional advice if the symptoms do not clear in a few days, or do not respond to simple measures.

In any urinary or kidney disorder avoid fluoridated water.

Barley water is healing, especially to the urinary system. For recipe see Cystitis. Take half a teacupful three times daily. Barley is rich in minerals and in vitamin B, is nutritious and tonic. Infrequent passing of urine will be helped, in most instances, by uva ursi tea, buchu leaves or clivers, more particularly when backache is present.

Take a normal infusion of either tea three times daily in wineglassful doses. Abbott's Parsley Piert pills or Buchu herbs, and Roberts' Buchu Backache compound, will be very helpful, as will Heath & Heather's Backache tablets, which contain both uva ursi and buchu. If these remedies have no effect, then the help of a practitioner must be sought.

Difficulty in passing urine in an older man could be due to an enlarged prostate gland.

Couch grass infusion will resolve many problems; make a normal infusion, taking a teacupful night and morning.

Children's' urinary problems often respond well to a combination of corn silk and marshmallow root. Prepare by simmering ½ *oz* (12.5g) of marshmallow root in 1 pint (0.5 litre) of boiling water for fifteen minutes and combining this with a teacupful of water to which two teaspoonfuls of corn silk have been added. See Children's' Ailments for dosage.

Uterine Disorders

The range of disorders which can cause problems really must have professional diagnosis and treatment. Herbal practitioners have a good range of remedies to dispense for many of these conditions.

Raspberry leaves have been mentioned in connection with pregnancy; the tea can be taken regularly at times other than during pregnancy for its tonic, astringent action, strengthening pelvic muscles. Its tonic properties will be reinforced if combined with equal quantities of gentian root and beth root. A wine glassful two or three times daily will be sufficient. Pain of the neuralgic, colicky type is relieved by wild yam; small doses taken frequently, hot, will be effective. Cramp is eased by warm infusions of cramp bark, or by agnus castus, which is available in tablet form or as a homoeopathic remedy.

General health must be attended to, a good diet, good posture, exercises to strengthen abdominal muscles, and warm or cold salt baths (hip baths) will all be helpful. Yoga is of benefit, but hard abdominal breathing must be avoided if there is a tendency to prolapse.

Tragically, hysterectomy is being recommended by the medical profession to younger and younger women.

Attention to the causes of uterine problems, early treatment with the right herbal remedies, supported by diet and exercise, has in many cases made surgery unnecessary.

Varicose Veins

Distended and unnaturally bulging veins in the legs arise from pressure on veins in the pelvis, caused by pregnancy, obesity or constipation, from poor circulation and weakened blood vessels, from too much standing, inadequate exercise and lowered general health. An hereditary tendency has also been noted, often evident in several generations.

Distilled witch-hazel applied daily, either painted over the veins and left to dry, or applied as a compress for an hour or so daily, will have a gently toning, astringent effect.

An infusion of tansy herb (1 teaspoonful to 1 teacupful of boiling water) as a lotion used in the same way, will strengthen the veins. A half-strength infusion can be taken in wineglassful doses twice daily. Marigold can be used similarly, both as a lotion and in wineglassful doses. It is prepared by adding two teaspoonsful of marigold petals to a cupful of boiling water, leaving it to infuse for ten minutes. If varicose eczema has developed, chickweed ointment will be found to soothe and heal.

Yarrow tea, taken cold in wineglassful doses, three times daily, will strengthen the veins. Yarrow is astringent, cleansing and healing, anti-haemorrhagic and antithrombotic; a most valuable and successful remedy for varicose veins. Rutin is a necessary adjunct to herbal teas, for strengthening smaller vessels. This is available as buckwheat, taken in infusion and in tablet form.

Exercises can help improve varicose veins: take brisk daily walks and spend a few minutes each morning and evening rising up on tiptoe and down again, up and down quickly six times, followed by rising on tiptoe and down to a squatting position six times; after a short pause go down into a squatting position and up on heels, six times.

Walking about the house on tiptoe also improves muscle tone in the legs. The exercises should be done barefoot.

Resting on a slant-board for half an hour daily will help the circulation and relieve gravity pressure on the veins.

Finally, try to avoid sitting with the legs crossed or with the legs folded underneath one. Try to sleep with the legs stretched out rather than bent.

Vertigo

A feeling that the room is spinning around one can be due to disease of the middle ear, a virus infection, disturbance in the nervous system or disorder of the liver. The cause should be found. The virus infection could be treated with infusion of wild indigo or by taking garlic oil capsules nightly.

General remedies to be tried, as opposed to specific ones, are wood betony and balm. A wine glassful of either, prepared in normal infusion, taken three or four times daily will often clear the milder cases due to nervous problems.

See also Tinnitus.

Warts and Verrucas
Sometimes due to a virus, warts may disappear quite quickly. Try the juice from dandelion stalks, a spot of castor oil, the orange juice from stalks of greater celandine (this can be acrid, do not let it spill onto the skin), lemon juice, or rub with garlic juice or a crushed garlic clove. The same treatment can be applied to verrucas.

Whitlow
Avery painful gathering at the base of, or down the side of, the fingernail. Foment with hot water, apply a poultice. Abbott's No.1 paste will draw the inflammation away.

Comfrey leaves applied hot with the liquid in which they have been infused will give relief. Comfrey ointment will help also. See also Abscesses.

Whooping Cough
This distressing condition can be treated successfully with herbal remedies. It would be wise, of course, to seek the help of a herbal practitioner. Keep the child in bed if the temperature is raised, or keep in a warm room. Give plenty of fruit juices, especially lemon juice in warm water with honey, or garlic honey. To prepare this, add a large clove of garlic, finely sliced, to 4oz (100g) of liquid honey, cover and leave to stand overnight. Add a teaspoonful to a cupful of hot water, to be sipped. A very useful remedy is a combination of one tablespoonful each of crushed linseed and thyme herb, 1 oz (25g) each of coltsfoot, white horehound and liquorice. Simmer the linseed and liquorice sticks (which have been peeled first) very gently in a covered pan for half an hour. Pour 1pint (0.5 litre) of boiling water over the other herbs, cover and leave to cool. Mix the two together, sieve and strain through a very fine

cloth or a paper coffee filter. The dose is a dessertspoonful for a child over five years old, two teaspoonfuls for a younger child and one teaspoonful for an infant. The dose can be given every four hours, with extra doses to relieve coughing as may be necessary.

Another useful remedy is equal quantities of angelica, hyssop and pennyroyal, 1oz (25g) of the mixture to 1 pint (0.5 litre) of cold water, brought to the boil then taken from the heat and left to stand for five minutes before straining.

The dose is as above.

Garlic is an excellent antiseptic and antibiotic, the old wives' cure for whooping cough which consisted of rubbing the soles of the feet with a cut clove of garlic has been proved effective by research. The antiseptic oil and other effective constituents have been shown to be carried to the lungs within half an hour of application to the feet.

Rub the chest with a good herbal liniment. Olbas oil is excellent. Keep the child off milk and dairy products.

Do not treat whooping cough without consulting a herbal practitioner.

Worms

It has been estimated that 200 million people throughout the world suffer from some form of intestinal parasite.

About thirty per cent of English children are affected at some time, mostly by threadworms. The parasites enter the body as larvae, developing fully within a few weeks and migrating to the intestines, liver, lungs or other parts of the body. The most common sources are infected and undercooked pork, beef or fish and insanitary drinking water. Dogs, cats and other pets may also be sources.

Threadworms are the cause of intense itching around the anus at night, resulting from the female migrating to lay eggs in the anus.

Garlic is an excellent antiseptic against parasites and should be used freely. Eat a clove of garlic each day (if you have the courage!) or failing that take three garlic oil capsules every night, and insert a capsule into the anus at night as a suppository. An infusion of quassia used as an enema will help to expel worms. Add 1 oz (25g) to 1pint (0.5 litres) of boiled water which has cooled for ten minutes.

Leave to stand until cool, and then strain through a fine cloth.

Warm the liquid to blood heat before use.

Do not eat meat or fish which is raw, undercooked or suspect. Wash salads and vegetables carefully. Change to a vegetarian diet, keep sugar to the minimum and eat plenty of carrots and pears. Molasses has been found to be successful in clearing tapeworm from the body; at least two teaspoonfuls should be taken daily. Pumpkin seeds may be eaten, but not by pregnant women.

Wounds

Keep the wound clean to avoid infection entering the bloodstream. Bathe with tepid water, apply crushed plantain leaves, or golden rod, or a pad of gauze soaked in distilled witch-hazel, or diluted tincture of marigold (one teaspoonful to a wineglassful of warm water), or an infusion of comfrey leaves. If there is any dirt in the wound do not stop the bleeding too quickly (unless loss of blood would be dangerous) as the blood will carry away most of the poisons. Add a few drops of tincture of myrrh to the liquid being used. Change the compress every twenty-four hours, soaking the bandage with plain warm water if it is adhering to the wound.

If the artery has been damaged the blood will be coming out in spurts, and firm pressure over the wound will be necessary, with clean fingers or a clean pad moistened with distilled witch-hazel.

2. First Aid Box and Holiday First Aid

In addition to the usual bandages, adhesive plasters, cotton wool, lint and scissors, the following will be found invaluable:

Antispasmodic tincture - for the relief of any type of nerve pain, taken in warm water, and also massaged over the painful area; to ease the effects of shock, for nausea and sickness; good as a quick tonic when feeling tired or dejected, and for nervousness.

Comfrey oil - to apply immediately to any bruises, sprains or injuries, will relieve the pain very quickly.

Bach Rescue Remedy - to counteract shock of any kind, can be taken every few minutes if necessary.

Distilled witch-hazel- a soothing gentle astringent to apply to bruises, sprains, insect bites, painful varicose veins, burns and sunburn, and as a compress on the eyes; will arrest haemorrhage.

Tincture of myrrh - an antiseptic, to apply well-diluted to wounds, bites, etc. It will smart. Apply neat to mouth ulcers.

Composition essence - taken in hot water to counteract chills and a feeling of chilliness; useful also for diarrhoea.

Elderflower, peppermint and composition – will ward off incipient colds, flu, etc.; taken in hot water will promote perspiration.

Chamomile flowers - to relieve nausea and sickness in adults and children; to calm the nerves.

Peppermint tea - for indigestion, will also ease headaches and relieve mental fatigue; useful for students at exam time.

Olbas oil (or some other herbal liniment) - to rub the chest in chesty colds or bronchitis, as an inhaler; to rub aching muscles.

Chickweed ointment - to heal wounds, lacerations, etc.; for burns, wasp and bee stings, to draw abscesses.

Oil of lavender - to repel insects, or to apply to insect stings; smoothed gently on the temples will ease migraine's headaches.

Slippery elm - a soothing drink for many digestive .and bowel disorders; useful also as a poultice.

Marshmallow root - very often gives effective relief to cystitis sufferers.

Raspberry leaves or Agrimony herb - to gently control diarrhoea, in both adults and children.

Powdered ginger - to ease painful flatulence and indigestion, a half-teaspoonful in a little hot water to be sipped slowly.

Holiday First Aid

One would not wish to appear to be a hypochondriac by carrying a large bagful of remedies 'just in case', but a few well-chosen items could prevent a holiday from being ruined. These would be selected from the domestic first aid box, and could well include:

Antispasmodic tincture - for nerve pains, shock, stomach upsets; to take to relieve sunstroke.

Distilled witch-hazel - for sunburn, burns, bruises, bleeding, insect bites.

Bach Rescue Remedy - to counteract shock, including sunstroke.

Composition essence - in hot water for chills; in cold water to help control diarrhoea.

Tincture of meadowsweet - in conjunction with composition essence will control stomach upsets and diarrhoea. Can be given to children.

Oil of lavender - to repel insects; to help relieve headaches.

Chamomile tea - for nausea; to calm the nerves.

Peppermint tea - to relieve indigestion; to ease headaches.

Olbas oil - to rub aching muscles; to rub the chest in colds and coughs; to inhale.

3. Nutrition

Herbal medicine can be most effective when used correctly, particularly when the right kinds of foods are eaten and the body does not have to contend with an excess of clogging, stodgy meals or with the innumerable chemical additives found in convenience foods. The changeover to a good diet may be made quickly by starting with a one or two-day fast followed by raw fruits and salads; cooked vegetables and vegetarian dishes together with wholemeal bread and cereals are then introduced within a few days. Alternatively, the change can be a more gradual one by changing one type of food at a time, such as changing from white bread to wholemeal, and so on. It is often found after one has adjusted to a fresh, whole foods diet that the incessant craving for sweet foods and chocolate vanishes completely.

Additionally, a higher level of health can be achieved and maintained by under-eating, by leaving the meal-table feeling pleasantly satisfied rather than full to bursting point.

It is only from the natural, raw foods grown on healthy soil that we can obtain real, lasting health and vitality.

Good health can be maintained, and moderate health improved, by a diet in which fifty per cent of food is raw (fruits, salads and vegetables, not raw meat and fish), and the remainder of the food consists of whole grains (bread, breakfast cereals, rice, barley, millet, etc.), natural cane sugar or honey in minimum quantities, mixed protein dishes of cheese, eggs, nuts, pulses and - if a vegetarian diet is not chosen - lean lamb and occasionally beef, fish, and naturally-reared fowl. Ill-health can in most cases be either partially or fully overcome by a completely raw-food diet, but this would wisely be carried out under the guidance of a practitioner experienced in fasting and strict dieting.

A suggested outline for a health-giving diet, which can be adjusted according to individual requirements, is as follows:

On rising - a drink of unsweetened fruit juice, sipped slowly (if grapefruit or lemon juice are taken they will be well-diluted and a little honey may be added).

Breakfast - some raw, fresh fruit, followed by stewed dried fruit if desired (prunes, dried fruit salad), either a wholegrain cereal (without added sugar) to which can be added nuts, sunflower seeds, sesame seeds, raisins, dates, or whole-wheat toast with vegetable margarine and honey, low-sugar marmalade or molasses.

Lunch - raw salad, either a little taken with packed lunch or a plate of fresh mixed salads, selected from watercress, lettuce, Chinese leaves or other greens, onions, grated raw carrot, celery, tomato, cucumber, radish, peppers, grated raw beetroot, small florets of raw cauliflower, as available, and dressed with vegetable oil and lemon juice, and some fresh chopped herbs sprinkled over.

Some cheese or other protein can be taken with the salad, and it can be accompanied by whole-wheat bread or crisp bread.

Evening - start with a piece of melon, small green salad or half grapefruit. This may be followed with home-made soup in cold weather. Choose a protein dish as a main course, with three or more conservatively-cooked vegetables. A fruit dish makes a satisfying dessert – fresh fruit, fruit salad, crumble, stewed or baked fruit, fruit jelly (made with agar-agar, the vegetarian gelatine), or natural yogurt with some honey and fruit added if desired.

Drinks between meals can be fruit juices, herb teas, *Vecon,* Yeastrel, weak China, Earl Grey or Luaka tea (all low in tannin), Dandelion coffee or other coffee substitute, Slippery elm or Barmene.

A few books which discuss diet in detail, and which give practical and mostly uncomplicated guidance for following a sensible and enjoyable diet, are given in the book list.

There are many more books available on the subject, and plenty of books on vegetarian diet.

THE END

Made in the USA
Coppell, TX
29 May 2023